D0192489

How to
Sleep
Soundly
Tonight

250 Simple and Natural Ways
to Prevent Sleeplessness

Barbara L. Heller

STOREY
BOOKS

Schoolhouse Road
Pownal, Vermont 05261

*The mission of Storey Communications is to serve our customers
by publishing practical information that encourages personal independence
in harmony with the environment.*

This publication is intended to provide educational information for the reader on the covered subject. It is not intended to take the place of personalized medical counseling, diagnosis, and treatment from a trained health professional.

Edited by Deborah Balmuth and Karen Levy
Cover design by Leslie Constantino
Cover photograph ©Matthias Kulka, The Stock Market
Text design by Susan Bernier and Jennifer Jepson Smith
Text production by Jennifer Jepson Smith
Line drawing on pages vi and 180 by Paul Hoffman
Indexed by Eileen M. Clawson

Printed in the United States by R.R. Donnelley
10 9 8 7 6 5 4 3 2

Library of Congress Cataloging-in-Publication Data

Heller, Barbara L.
    How to sleep soundly tonight: 250 simple and natural ways to prevent sleeplessness / by Barbara L. Heller.
        p.   cm.
    ISBN 1-58017-314-4 (alk. paper)
    1. Sleep — Popular works. 2. Sleep disorders — Popular works. I. Title.
RA786.H45 2001
616.8'498—dc21   00-052220
                                                             CIP

Table of Contents

— To my daughter, Rebecca —

Acknowledgments

Heartfelt thanks to my wonderful circle of supporters: Phyllis Heller, Paula Kephart, Susan Maguire, Suzanne Massa, Zach Rosen, Barbara Ruchames, Bob Ruchames, Tess Taft, and Irene Zahava. I appreciate your friendship and your generous assistance. Thanks also to Gretchen Adams, Melissa Collins, Jessie Eisenberg, Kathy Grandison, Kristen Stiles, and Janet Wilson for your suggestions. I love public libraries and greatly appreciate the enthusiastic assistance of the reference desk staff at the Binghamton Public Library and my friendly and helpful local librarian, Ramona Bogart, at the Afton Free Library.

I am indebted to all those who have shared their sleep challenges with me in psychotherapy, during workshops, and through the "Women Sharing Sleep Stories" survey. I have also learned a tremendous amount from the written work of the premier sleep researcher and educator Dr. William Dement.

Thanks to the entire team at Storey, especially my editors, Deborah Balmuth and Karen Levy.

And, as always, my gratitude to my family: my sleep partner, Alan, and my daughter, Rebecca. Although it has been a challenging summer, I will remember how many times you each reread the manuscript. I cherish your love and support.

Preface

A night of refreshing sleep is one of life's sweet pleasures. Deep and restful sleep provides the foundation for our active lives and gives us energy to appreciate joyful times. Simply put, good sleep prepares us for great days.

As a psychotherapist and educator for the past two decades, I have spoken with many sleep-challenged clients, students, colleagues, and friends. And I have experienced periods of sleep problems, as well. I know that most sleep troubles caused by stress, travel, illness, and physical changes are temporary. For occasional or periodic insomnia, self-help strategies can provide relief.

This book includes summaries of current research and suggestions for how to get a good night's sleep. Read on to:

- ★ Identify physical and cultural obstacles to sleep
- ★ Alter your negative attitudes about sleep
- ★ Assess your own sleep problems
- ★ Learn habits that enhance sleep
- ★ Dream up an inviting sleep environment
- ★ Learn how to relax with deep breathing, meditation, yoga, visualizations, and other calming techniques
- ★ Discover natural herbal and homeopathic sedatives
- ★ Enjoy recipes for tranquil herbal baths, sleep pillows, and room sprays
- ★ Decide whether or not to consult a professional

What do you have to lose? Certainly, no more of your precious slumber. And what do you have to gain? Deep and restful sleep and the health and energy it creates. With this book on your nightstand, you'll sleep soundly every night!

Barbara L. Heller, M.S.W.

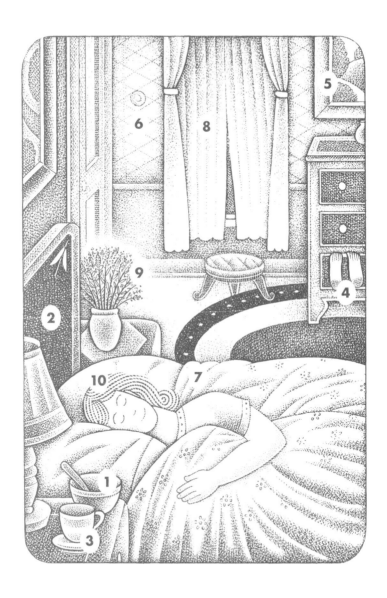

Ten Things You Can Do Today to Sleep Soundly Tonight

1. Have a bowl of cereal or a slice of bread 40 minutes before bedtime.

2. Make sure your bed isn't in a direct line with a door or a bathroom. Don't place your bed under beams and don't store items underneath your bed.

3. Drink a cup of chamomile tea or try another safe herbal sedative.

4. Put on warm, fluffy socks or place a hot-water bottle near your feet.

5. Decorate with peaceful artwork.

6. Set the temperature to 65°F (18°C).

7. Indulge in soft sheets, fluffy pillows, and a plush comforter.

8. Hang room-darkening curtains to shield bright streetlights.

9. Inhale the scent of lavender from a lavender-scented sleep pillow placed between your regular pillow and pillowcase.

10. After you are tucked in, count your blessings, count your breaths, or count backward from 100.

1

How and Why We Sleep

If you heard about a new product guaranteed to increase health and productivity, would you purchase it? If the local gym promoted exercise classes that ensured improvement in your mood and behavior, would you sign up? Well, there is an activity, which can be practiced almost anywhere and at no cost, that can provide these benefits and more. The activity is *sleep,* and it can reward you with increased health and energy, and a fresh perspective.

Sleep is the physiological function that helps nourish our mind, body, and soul. It is essential for good health and upbeat spirits. During slumber, we experience memory consolidation and physical restoration and growth. Sleep also helps us recover from illnesses and enhances our resistance to disease.

Sound sleep can greatly improve our daily lives. When we wake from restful, refreshing sleep, we feel renewed and ready to face the day ahead. In addition, being well-rested enhances our mood, our ability to learn, and our coping skills. It also increases our capacity for communication, creativity, and concentration. When we increase the quality of our sleep, we age more gracefully.

"[People] cannot long survive without air, water, and sleep."

THOMAS SZASZ, M.D.

Make Sleep a Star

Get more sleep! This is not often a rallying cry, or the topic of fantasies. Although other bedroom activity is given more press, better sleep gives you more energy, improves your mood, makes you less prone to accidents

How Much Is Enough?

On a daily basis, when you get a sufficient amount of sleep:

★ You don't need to rely on an alarm clock to wake up.

★ You feel rested and alert.

★ You don't doze off while watching TV or while sitting and reading.

★ You don't fall asleep in public places, such as movie theaters or school classes.

★ You don't get drowsy in a car — either as a driver or as a passenger.

★ You don't feel so tired that it interferes with your daily activities.

and less irritable, and increases your life span. And those benefits may also make you feel more romantic.

Often, we take sleep for granted. It is only when we are sleep deprived that those around us are most apt to notice. Family members, friends, or coworkers may comment, "Seems like you got up on the wrong side of the bed this morning." In some circles, being exhausted is worn like a badge of honor.

The National Commission on Sleep Disorders asserts, "America is seriously sleep deprived, with serious consequences." Lack of sleep decreases productivity, effectiveness, concentration, decision-making abilities, and physiological immunity. Consistently being deprived of sleep can increase the severity of diabetes, obesity, hypertension, and age-related disorders. Sleepiness has been implicated in accidents on the road, in the air, in hospitals, and at nuclear power plants. When sleep deprivation is combined with driving, the results can be as dangerous and as fatal as those of drunk driving.

On the other hand, sound sleep provides physical, psychological, and spiritual benefits. William Dement, M.D., Ph.D., a leading authority on sleep and sleep disorders, claims, "Healthy sleep has been empirically proven to be the single most important determinant in predicting longevity, more influential than diet, exercise, or heredity."

Sleep may also be crucial to spiritual well-being. Clark Strand, author and former Zen monk, ranks sleep number one of seven practices that will help you live more joyfully every day. He says, "Sleep is indispensable for the experience of 'enoughness' in our lives. The basis for clear awareness during our waking hours, it determines more than any other factor the overall quality of our days." Give sleep top billing and it will prepare you for peak performance.

The Rhythm of Sleep

The American Heritage Dictionary defines sleep as "A natural, periodic state of rest for the mind and body, in which the eyes usually close and consciousness is completely or partially lost, so that there is a decrease in bodily movement and responsiveness to external stimuli." Although the adjective *sleepy* can be used to mean inactive, and that may seem true to an observer, sleep is really an active state.

There are two basic types of sleep. Nonrapid eye movement (NREM) sleep, as its name suggests, is characterized by little or no eye movement. Physical changes that occur during NREM sleep include the slowing down of breathing and heart rate. NREM sleep occurs in four progressively deeper stages. When we initially fall asleep, we enter stage 1 REM sleep. We spend the longest period of our sleep time in stage 2 NREM sleep. The last two NREM stages, 3 and 4, mark our deepest levels of sleep but make up only about 20 percent of our total sleep time.

Rapid eye movement (REM) sleep is when most dreaming occurs. It is marked by a distinctive shifting of the eyes that can be detected by watching the sleeper's face. Most people experience four to six REM periods of increasing length during any given night. Paradoxically, REM sleep is both the most active and the most inactive sleep stage. People experience many physiological changes, including increased blood pressure, pulse, and respiration; erections; and a rise in body temperature. But during REM sleep, the muscles are temporarily paralyzed. This sleep paralysis is a form of physiological self-protection from the potential danger and damage we could experience if we were to act out our dreams.

There is a rhythmic pattern to sleep. During a normal night, adults cycle between REM sleep and NREM sleep in regular patterns. REM sleep occurs approximately every 90 minutes. During this cycle, people fall into progressively deeper stages of NREM sleep and then cycle back through the stages until they enter REM sleep again.

The Biological Clock

Although lacking a numbered dial and moving hands, an internal biological clock regulates all our major bodily functions. A tiny cluster of brain cells near the optic nerves, described as our internal biological clock, orchestrates the intricate cyclical connections of temperature, hormones, mood, appetite, alertness, and other physiological functions.

The activities governed by our body's clock follow a pattern that takes about 24

"We eat, think, exercise, wake up, and sleep best when we heed the rhythm of our inner clock."

DR. WILLIAM DEMENT

Anticipation as an Alarm Clock

Will stating your intention to get up at 6 A.M. allow you to discard your morning siren? Some people awake at a specific time just by thinking about it. German researchers found that subjects who planned to wake up at a specified time experienced a surge of a "timekeeping" hormone approximately one hour prior to their planned waking. If you try this at home, set a backup alarm for 10 minutes later than the appointed time, in case your internal clock doesn't arouse you.

hours and is called circadian rhythm (derived from the Latin *circa*, meaning around, and *ðian/ðies*, meaning day). Scientists have found that the internal clock has a tendency to run from 10 minutes to more than an hour longer than 24 hours. What are the implications of this schedule?

Our internal clock regulates our level of alertness, so to be healthy and attentive we need to coordinate our body clock with that of the cultural timepiece and calendar. Light is the major external factor that influences this natural rhythm. The brain also relies on social contact, regular meal and sleep times,

Optimal Timing

The relatively new field of chronotherapy is based on the belief that we can enhance health by timing medical interventions to coincide with our circadian rhythms. Researchers know that there are times of day when humans are most prone to certain conditions. For example, more heart attacks and strokes occur in the morning than at any other time of day. It may be possible to synchronize medical treatments with our biological clocks in order to optimize the effects of medications and medical procedures.

and other outside influences to keep it on a 24-hour schedule. Insufficient light and lack of sleep can disturb circadian rhythms. The best ways to keep in sync with our internal clocks are to maintain consistent sleep schedules and get daily doses of early-morning light and evening darkness.

The National Sleep Debt

The average adult needs seven to nine hours of sleep to function well. This varies by age, gender, and personal physiology. Nearly one-third of Americans gets by on six and a half hours of sleep or less. Only 35 percent of adults sleep the recommended eight hours or more per night during the work-week. Since more than 50 percent of Americans get up at 6 A.M. or earlier, lights-out for most adults should be before 10 P.M. Skimping on sleep is a relatively recent cultural development. Prior to electricity, people rose at dawn and went to sleep soon after sunset. At the turn of the last century, the average American slept about nine hours a night.

One of the most important measures of adequate sleep is your level of alertness during the day. Sleep experts agree that most people need from 40 to 90 minutes more sleep than they get in order to be fully alert and to improve their overall health and performance.

When our sleep cycles are curtailed, either physiologically or by choice, we become sleep deprived. Sleep educators have coined the term "sleep debt" to describe how sleep deprivation works. "Each of us maintains a personal sleep bank account," explains James Maas, Ph.D., Cornell University professor and author of *Power Sleep*. "Any sleep you get is a deposit or an asset; any hour of wakefulness is a withdrawal or a debit.

Most people need to deposit at least eight hours of sleep in the account to cancel the sleep debt incurred by 16 hours of continuous alertness." Sleep debt is cumulative. The catch-22 is that trying to catch up on lost sleep — by sleeping more than two hours later than usual — may actually cause subsequent sleep problems.

Morning Larks and Night Owls

The times that you go to sleep and wake up are important. Are you a "morning lark" or a "night owl"? Larks function best in the early hours, while owls are still sleeping; the optimal time for owls, naturally, is at night. It seems likely that larks penned the proverbs "The early bird catches the worm" and "Early to bed and early to rise makes a man healthy, wealthy, and wise." Research suggests that only about 20 percent of the population is truly at either extreme, but it is helpful to be aware of your own tendencies. At what time of day are you most alert? Use that time to tackle creative or difficult tasks. Allot downtime for less challenging activities.

"You eat, in dreams, the custard of the day."

ALEXANDER POPE

The Meaning of Dreams

Most of us dream as much as two hours a night. Our inner movies are rich with mental pictures and emotions. Sometimes we awake on the edge of a dream, barely holding on to the fuzzy vision. Other times, we wake up with a racing heart and nightmare images. Some people say that they never dream, but they do, they just don't remember.

What is the function of these elusive illusions? Throughout history, cultures have searched for personal and communal meanings for their dreamscapes. Various theories emphasize the purpose of dreaming as a means to preserve sleep, to reveal something to ourselves, to conceal ideas from our conscious mind, to solidify memory and problem solving, and to clean out the day's debris.

Psychological Function

Dreams serve a psychological function. They are "the royal road to the unconscious," as Sigmund Freud wrote more than a hundred years ago. Freud believed that the latent meaning of dreams focused on personal impulses, or "the imaginary gratification of unconscious wishes," which were usually repressed sexual feelings. Carl Jung theorized that dreams are constructed not only from personal images but also from archetypes, the symbols of a larger collective unconscious. His dream interpretations drew from mythology, religion, spirituality, and common cultural symbols.

Physiological Function

Dreaming also serves a physiological function. Modern neuroscientists postulate that dreams are a result of the random firing of neurons. During our dream state, we rid ourselves of unneeded memories; in essence, dreaming acts as a self-cleaning mechanism of the brain. The more studying, learning, and problem solving we do during the day, the longer we spend in REM sleep and dreaming. Growing children spend a large proportion of their sleep time in the REM stage. One study of older people revealed that those who had the most REM sleep also had the most active minds and the best memory recall.

Insight and Understanding

Do you believe that dreams can help you better understand your life and the world around you? If so, you can use your dreams

"I remember my dreams every morning, but if I don't write them down, they flit away. They go back to their own world again."

AMY TAN, AUTHOR

as a springboard for inner exploration. Gayle Delaney, Ph.D., author of *All About Dreams,* asks, "To what uses can you put the insights you have gained by noting the metaphors in your dream that relate to your waking life?"

Can Dreams Forecast the Future?

Some mind/body practitioners believe that dreams can be an early warning signal of disease. One Russian study found that dreams sometimes pinpointed an illness prior to diagnosis. But dreams of illness can also be a sign of our anxieties. In his book *The Promise of Sleep,* Dr. William Dement recounts a vivid personal example. He dreamed that he was diagnosed with lung cancer. At the time, he was a heavy cigarette smoker and his dream was the impetus for him to quit smoking. For Dr. Dement, the dream foretold a possible but not a certain outcome. He now believes that dream gave him a second chance at life.

"I think that every creative impulse that a working writer or artist of any sort has, comes out of the dark old country where dreams come from."

ANNE RIVERS SIDDONS

2

How Sleep Changes over Time

We face different sleep challenges throughout our life cycle. Gender, age, responsibilities, and even time of year can affect how well we sleep. Infants and young children experience the longest and deepest periods of sleep. When adolescence approaches, sleep is disturbed by a growing number of cultural and physical obstacles.

Daily demands at school, work, and home increase as we age, seeming to conspire against our getting a full night's sleep. Women's sleep can be challenged by hormonal fluctuations during the reproductive years. Aging men and women experience physiological and cultural changes that make consistent sleep more difficult.

Sleeping Children

Babies sure sleep a lot — but not always when their parents would like them to. The average newborn sleeps from 15 to 20 hours in a 24-hour cycle. Often that sleep is broken up into spurts lasting from two to four hours. Vicky Lansky, in her book *Getting Your Child to Sleep*, explains that during a baby's first six months of life, sleep patterns are largely a reflection of biological development. Simply put, infants sleep when they are tired and wake when they are hungry.

But their sleep patterns and difficulties, such as evening awakenings, bed-wetting, and nightmares, have more effect on their caretakers. Lansky goes on to reassure new parents, "Whether or not your baby is a good sleeper is not a reflection of your parenting skills or of the baby's goodness. Try not to equate sleep with happiness or superiority."

Night-Lights

The advisability of the old parental tool against night fears, the night-light, is being questioned. A preliminary study conducted at the University of Pennsylvania concluded that young children who are exposed to light while they sleep are five times more likely to develop nearsightedness (myopia) than are those who sleep in the dark.

Although two follow-up studies were unable to duplicate these results, researchers point out that animal studies have proved a link between eye development and the cycles of light and dark. Therefore, some experts advise parents to minimize their children's nighttime exposure to artificial light.

Infants' and toddlers' sleep patterns naturally change over time as the need for sleep gradually decreases. Young children sleep from 10 to 12 hours a night; this amount lessens when they discontinue regular daytime naps. Parents need to understand and adapt to these phases. You can also enhance your child's sleep (as well as your own) by providing a sleep-inducing environment and reinforcing positive nighttime habits.

At-Home Parents

If you are home with children during the day, nap when they do. Don't use their downtime as a chance to catch up on your chores. If you do, you'll just end up exhausted at the end of the day.

Soothe, Don't Stimulate

Does your baby love Bach? Music is a magical reinforcement for parents with cranky children. Lullabies soothe both babies and their caretakers. Supplement those simple songs with classical compositions and recordings of ocean waves and other sounds of nature to invite sleep into a child's bedroom. Many neonatal units play tapes of lullabies softly enhanced with the sound of human heartbeats to calm crying infants and put them to sleep.

On the other hand, television may act as a stimulant. Children who watch a lot of it, especially near bedtime, are more likely to resist going to sleep and exhibit more sleep problems. Study director Judith Owens, M.D., M.P.H., of Brown University says, "A lot of parents don't make the connection. They think if TV is sedating for adults, it is for kids, too. Some TV in the evening is fine. Just don't make it part of your child's bedtime routine." Loud music; interaction with older, more active siblings; and computer use should also be limited.

Establish Evening Routines

Comic-strip child Dennis the Menace once complained, "Just because I'm sleepy doesn't mean I want to go to bed." Children do not

"Good-bye, dear child. I wish you good sleep and good digestion. I don't know anything better to desire for those I love."

LOUISE HONORINE DE CHOISEUL, 18TH-CENTURY FRENCH WRITER

equate tiredness with sleep; adults must teach them to make the association. Throughout childhood, bedtime can be a relaxing, winding-down time for both parents and children, providing a special time to connect. Expecting an evening routine helps children prepare for bedtime. Parenting experts agree that predictability makes children's lives more manageable. A bath followed by storytelling or book reading, then cuddling with a comforting nighttime companion, such as a favorite teddy bear or blanket, will help your child doze off for the night.

However, the time after the "final" good nights often becomes a nightmare. How should you respond to a child's third cry of "I want another drink of water"? Pediatric researchers recommend a behavioral technique to effectively deal with this frustrating habit. Children are issued a "pass" for one drink or one trip to the bathroom after lights-out. Setting clear limits and rules in a loving and understanding context will help make bedtime more pleasurable for everyone.

Tired Teenagers

Adolescents are the most in debt — sleep debt, that is. During the teen years, lifestyle choices often compete with physiological needs. Sleep loss negatively affects how teens learn and how they perform academically. Studies show that to function well, teens need 9 to 10 hours of sleep a night, but most average only 6. It is important for parents and teachers to realize that when teenagers "sleep in," it is generally not because they are lazy. They need the extra hours to refuel. The National Sleep Foundation reports that 60 percent of children under the age of 18 complain of feeling tired during the day.

Teens' sleep patterns are biological, not just cultural. It is estimated that between 80 and 90 percent of young people are night owls. Sleep researchers say that adolescents experience a natural physiological change in their circadian rhythm to a phase-delayed inner clock. Even though they may be tired during the day, their ability to sleep shuts down at around 7:30 P.M. and doesn't turn on again for hours. This means that the night owl schedule that the average teen desires has a physiological basis.

Teenagers often try to catch up on lost sleep during the weekend, but there is a downside to this habit. Waking 2 to 3 hours later on Saturday and Sunday than they do on school mornings can make it harder for teens to rise when they go back to their weekday routines.

School schedules also conflict with teens' natural sleep rhythm. More than one study has shown that teenagers who start school two hours later than usual perform better on academic tests. School districts with later start times report better grades and fewer discipline problems. In addition, sleep deprivation increases teenagers' chances of automobile accidents and may predispose them to sleep disorders. Furthermore, research shows that sleep-deprived teens are more prone to become drug users or to act out aggressively.

When we add the natural night owl tendency of teens to an incredible array of activities competing for their attention, we understand why teens often cut sleep short. Many adolescents juggle a full schedule of school and homework, a part-time job, sports, and other extracurricular activities.

Homes are also overflowing with enticing games and activities. In the past, kids may have spent a few extra minutes in the evening with a book and a flashlight under the bedcovers; now they have high-tech alternatives. More than one parent has "caught" an adolescent chatting on-line in the wee hours. The National Sleep Foundation warns that studying and playing computer games before bed are arousing, as is trying to sleep with a computer or TV flickering in the bedroom. Therefore, parents may need to set limits for their children's sake.

Jack and Jill Went . . . to Sleep

The nightly cycles of REM and NREM sleep are similar in both sexes, but women and men are prone to different sleep challenges. Some experts believe that women just need more sleep than men do. "If a man

"Who does not like to fall asleep with the rain beating on the roof and the wind rubbing the outer walls, while oneself is dry and warm in a comfortable bed?"

SENA JETER NASLUND,
AHAB'S WIFE

and woman keep the same hours, the woman is likely to be sleep deprived," say Allen Frances, M.D., and Michael B. First, M.D., authors of *Your Mental Health: A Layman's Guide to the Psychiatrist's Bible.*

Women are twice as likely as men to have difficulty falling asleep or staying asleep, and a larger percentage of women report not feeling refreshed upon waking. Whether maiden, mother, or elder, a woman can be sleep challenged by hormonal fluctuations. More than half the women who responded to one national survey reported having sleep disruptions for at least two or three days of every menstrual cycle. According to the same survey, premenstrual symptoms disturbed the sleep of at least 25 percent of women in the week before their periods.

Pregnancy is a very tiring experience. Almost 80 percent of pregnant women complain that their sleep is worse than before their pregnancy. Morning sickness, leg cramps, heartburn, and an increase in fetal size and movement all interfere with sleep. The lack of sleep seems like preparation for parenting a newborn: A new mother may lose as many as 700 hours of sleep before her baby's first birthday.

Menopause presents its own sleep challenges. Fluctuating estrogen levels throw off a woman's internal temperature gauge. Hot flashes and their sleep-time equivalent, night sweats, plague many menopausal women. Hot flashes followed by chills after the sweat evaporates can wake a woman during the night; she may need to change her drenched nightgown or bedding. Mood swings and heart palpitations can also keep women awake during this phase.

Compared with women, men snore more and are eight times more likely to develop sleep apnea, a serious sleep disorder associated with an increased risk of heart attack and stroke (see page 40). Prostate problems, which are common in aging men, contribute to increased nighttime awakenings to urinate. Men also have a much higher rate of REM sleep behavior disorder, a rare but serious problem in which a sleeper acts out his dreams, potentially hurting himself or others.

Parents of young children, caretakers of elderly and infirm parents, people who work outside the home and are responsible for the majority of household tasks, and those who work long hours may become victims of the cultural aspect of sleep deprivation. Many people, women especially, curtail sleep in an attempt to accomplish it all.

Sleep-Challenged Seniors

True or false? Senior citizens don't need as much sleep as they did when they were younger. The correct answer is false.

It is a myth that the elderly don't *need* as much sleep, but it is true that they don't seem to *get* as much. Why? The American Sleep Disorders Foundation says, "Aging makes sleep more fragile, even in healthy older people." Although seniors may have fewer demands on their time, they face additional physiological obstacles to sleep.

The elderly experience more fragmented sleep. The average 60-year-old awakens more than 20 times a night; a young person, half as many times. Many of these awakenings are brief "microarousals" that the person is not conscious of, yet they contribute to daytime fatigue. The National Institutes of Health estimates that sleep disturbances affect more than 50 percent of people over the age of 65 living at home and two-thirds of the seniors in long-term-care facilities.

Seniors also get less deep (stages 3 and 4 NREM) sleep. In addition, sleep problems are often a side effect of other illnesses and conditions that become more common as we age, including arthritis, osteoporosis, prostate problems, ulcers, heartburn, chronic pain, depression, and grief.

But the good news is that seniors' sleep can be more satisfying. Health headlines herald that "Psychotherapy Tops Sleeping Pills in Research Study of Late-Life Insomnia." An important study, which compared counseling and medication as insomnia treatments for those over 65, found that cognitive-behavioral therapy was the most effective sleep aid. Therapy focused on basic sleep habits, such as going to bed only when you're tired, not watching TV in bed, and getting up at the same time every day.

Surprisingly, those who participated in only the group counseling sessions sustained more improvement in their sleep patterns than the group receiving a combination of medication and counseling. These results are quite significant, since the majority of prescriptions for sleep medications are given to seniors.

Studies have shown that seniors can be soothed to sleep with aromatherapy, music, or acupressure. Daily exercise is also important. A 1988 Gallup poll found that active retirees had fewer sleep problems than those who were sedentary. In addition, many sleep educators encourage seniors to nap to supplement the hours they sleep.

Seasons of Sleep

Just as sleep patterns change over the life cycle, they also shift with the season. The new year may call for resolutions, but many of us don't have the energy to stick with them — we are too tired from limited daylight and the after-effects of the holidays. The lack of sunlight affects some people so severely that they develop seasonal affective disorder, a form of clinical depression.

Ahhh, but then the warm days of spring finally arrive. Sleep may beckon you until . . . daylight saving time. Statistically, the one thing that most affects our seasonal sleep cycle is setting the clocks forward an hour. Analyses show an increase in death rates and traffic accidents for the week following the "lost hour." The time shift also negatively affects international stock markets. On the Monday following "spring forward," declines are two to five times larger than on the average Monday.

Stanley Coren, in his book *Sleep Thieves*, presents a convincing argument when he says, "Sixty minutes more in bed seems like a small investment, but it is clear that in our current sleep-debt-ridden state, it does pay large dividends." You can reap the reward by scheduling extra sleep the week after turning the clocks forward in the spring.

Next comes good old summertime, when the living is easy. Many people feel more energetic and stay active longer during the period of increased sunlight, but others lose sleep as a result of heat and humidity. Vacation sleep can be delicious, but it may also be challenged by the need to adapt to travel and new timetables.

Autumn completes the cycle. Again, we readjust our sleep patterns to accommodate

Spring Allergies

In the spring, new hopes and activities abound, but these may be accompanied by new allergens. Seasonal allergies and the medications that treat them can rob us of sleep. Over-the-counter allergy remedies may contain antihistamines, decongestants, or a combination of the two. Antihistamines (see page 175) may cause negative side effects along with drowsiness, while decongestants that contain pseudoephedrine can elevate blood pressure and pulse rate and cause difficulty falling asleep.

school and work schedules. Although we gain an hour of sleep when we turn the clocks back in the fall, our energy may wane as the hours of darkness increase. Many people also report sleep loss as they begin preparing for the holidays.

Do you notice any changes in your sleep patterns throughout the year? Awareness of the seasonal sleep sequence may help you identify and rectify sleep challenges before they become crises.

"I wake up in the morning torn between the desire to save the world and to enjoy the world."

E.B. WHITE

3

Do You Have a Sleep Problem?

Do you find it hard to fall asleep, your mind racing with thoughts and worries from the day? Do you toss and turn, rouse often, and wake up tired? Do you drag through your day with low energy? If you experience any of these symptoms, you are not alone.

According to the National Sleep Foundation, two-thirds of all Americans report a recognizable sleep problem. It's estimated that nearly 95 percent of sleep disorders go undiagnosed and untreated. When sleep disorders are not properly treated, they can become serious.

If your inability to get a good night's sleep is persistent, if you suffer from daytime fatigue, if your housemates complain about your snoring or other sleep habits, or if you exhibit any of the symptoms of the disorders described below, it's time for a medical evaluation. In addition to receiving a full physical exam, you may be referred for a sleep study at a specialized center. Consult your health-care practitioner for assessment and treatment.

Many physical, psychological, and cultural obstacles prevent us from getting consistently refreshing sleep. This chapter will help you assess your sleep problems and habits with a sleep diary. It also describes the signs and symptoms of common sleep disorders and lists diseases, conditions, and attitudes that can negatively affect your sleep.

Keep a Sleep Diary

The first step to improving your sleep is to keep track of your sleep patterns and your level of satisfaction with the quantity and quality of your slumber. This assessment can help you choose possible remedies for refreshing sleep. It can also be valuable to your work with a health-care practitioner if self-help strategies are not potent enough to resolve your sleep problem.

Describe the Problem

Answer the following questions to assess your overall sleep problem.

1. How long have you had trouble sleeping?
2. Is it a problem every night?
3. How do your sleep difficulties affect your daily functioning?
4. What current changes or stresses are you experiencing?
5. Does your sleep differ on the weekends or while you are on vacation?

"I have three phobias which, could I mute them, would make my life as slick as a sonnet, but as dull as ditch water: I hate to go to bed, I hate to get up, and I hate to be alone."

TALLULAH
BANKHEAD

Assess Your Nightly Sleep

Write down your answers to the following questions every day for two weeks.

1. What time did you go to bed last night?
2. About how long did it take you to get to sleep?
3. Did you awaken during the night? If so, how many times? What did you do when you awoke (stayed in bed, went to the bathroom, had a cigarette, ate something, worried)? How long did it take you to get back to sleep?
4. How many hours in total did you sleep last night?
5. What time did you get up this morning?
6. Did you use an alarm clock?
7. On a scale of 1 (still tired) to 5 (refreshed), how did you feel when you woke up?
8. Did you nap today? If so, when and for how long?
9. Did you take any medications today? How much alcohol or caffeinated substances did you consume? Did you smoke cigarettes?

10. What did you eat today? When and for how long did you exercise?

11. How did you feel today? Were you anxious, depressed, irritable, forgetful, or accident-prone?

12. On a scale of 1 (drowsy or fatigued) to 5 (energetic), how would you rate your functioning during the day?

Common Sleep Disorders

Dr. William Dement states, "My most significant finding is that ignorance is the worst sleep disorder of them all." Health professionals have classified more than 80 sleeping and waking disorders. Following are some of the most common ones.

Insomnia

Insomnia, the inability to get to sleep or stay asleep, is the most common sleep problem. Sleep-disorder professionals differentiate among many types of insomnia on the basis of their physical and psychological causes and how long the problem persists. Many insomniacs can be helped with a combination of natural treatments. For others, the debilitating cycle of chronic insomnia may be broken with the short-term use of prescription sleep medications.

Sleep Apnea

This disorder affects 20 to 30 million Americans. It is literally a breath-stopping disorder in which sleepers may snore and gasp as they stop and start breathing many times during the night. Sleep apnea is more prevalent in older, overweight men who snore, but it affects women and younger people as well. The condition is associated with high blood pressure and other heart problems.

Sufferers may find relief with a continuous positive air pressure (CPAP) machine, which is worn during sleep to combat breathlessness by forcing air into the nose. Other treatments include medications that aid proper nighttime breathing and behavior modifications, such as weight loss and limiting alcohol intake before bed. In extreme cases, physicians may recommend surgery to remove or shrink excess mouth and throat tissue.

Narcolepsy

Narcolepsy is a chronic neurological disorder that tends to run in families and produces excessive daytime sleepiness, daytime "sleep attacks," and cataplexy, or a loss of muscle control often brought on by strong emotions. Obviously, this disorder can be quite disruptive. A combination of prescription medications (usually stimulants and/or antidepressants) and behavior changes (including the judicious use of napping) can help alleviate some of the narcoleptic's challenges.

Restless Leg Syndrome

This condition is characterized by distinctly uncomfortable physical reactions and sensations — creeping, crawling, tingling, or pain — that disturb sleep but may also occur during daytime activities. Sufferers may find temporary relief through movement, massage, or showering. Periodic leg movement, a related syndrome, is characterized by leg twitching and jerking during the night that is severe enough to consistently wake the sleeper or a partner.

Other Problems

Some other conditions that may disturb sleep include sleepwalking, night terrors, delayed-sleep-phase syndrome, night eating syndrome, REM sleep behavior disorder, and bruxism (teeth grinding).

Medical Conditions and Medications

If you are sleeping poorly, a physical exam can help identify medical conditions and medications that are among the many known to be sleep thieves.

Medical Conditions That Affect Sleep

Insomnia can be a secondary effect of heart disease, allergies, asthma, diabetes, prostate problems, nutritional deficiencies, gastro-esophageal reflux, and sinus infections. In addition, the pain and stiffness of arthritis and fibromyalgia can cause people to awaken during the night. Premenstrual syndrome, pregnancy, and menopause may disrupt sleep, since hormonal fluctuations can play a major role in insomnia.

Heads Up to Relieve Heartburn

If heartburn and gastroesophageal reflux have been keeping you up at night, these remedies may help:

- ★ Try over-the-counter medications that block acid secretion.
- ★ Don't eat a full meal before bedtime.
- ★ Sleep with your upper body elevated (raise the head of your bed on wooden blocks or use extra pillows to prop you up).

There is also a high correlation between depression and insomnia. "There's no question that insomnia by itself will lead to depression. But the opposite is also true. About 80 to 90 percent of depressed patients have insomnia," reports David Neubauer, M.D., associate director of the Johns Hopkins University Sleep Disorder Center. Other emotional problems and psychological disorders, including anxiety and panic, seasonal affective disorder, and post-traumatic stress disorder, can curtail needed sleep.

Medications That Affect Sleep

Sleep disorders can be substance induced. Illegal drugs, especially cocaine and amphetamines, cause a host of sleeping problems, as do the socially sanctioned stimulants alcohol, tobacco, and coffee. Withdrawal from alcohol and nicotine can also cause insomnia. Many prescription medicines and over-the-counter remedies disturb sleep. If you are taking steroids; chemotherapy agents; diuretics; appetite suppressants; cold remedies; thyroid medications; antidepressants; or drugs for allergies, pain, asthma, a heart condition, or Parkinson's disease, read the package inserts or ask your pharmacist whether they may be contributing to your sleeplessness.

The effects of some medications are paradoxical. For example, antihistamines put some people to sleep but keep others awake. And the fact that something is "natural" doesn't mean it can't have negative side effects. Certain herbal formulas touted as tonics, energizers, or diet aids can rob you of desired sleep.

If you suspect that a medical condition or the medication you are taking is cutting into your sleep time, talk with your health-care professional. He or she can help by prescribing another medication or by changing the present dose or the time that it is taken.

Cheating Sleep: The National Pastime

Too many of us cheat ourselves of sleep as a way to cope with the conflicting demands of work, family, and personal needs. This deliberate sleep deprivation may be a precursor to involuntary insomnia and other health problems.

"But I have promises to keep, And miles to go before I sleep."

ROBERT FROST

On the Go

How often do you barter sleep for other activities? Is sleep on the bottom of your to-do list? Our individual choices and over-committed schedules often run counter to our physiology. One study found that 58 percent of Americans mistakenly believe that they can learn to function normally with 1 to 2 fewer hours of sleep than they need. "Sleep is the account we dip into when we are looking for time to do everything else," writes Andrea Van Steenhouse, Ph.D., in her book *A Woman's Guide to a Simpler Life.*

Too often, we are advised to give up sleep for other, supposedly more important activities or made to feel guilty if we regularly sleep the amount of time our bodies need. Headlines seem to proclaim, "Precious Little Time: Every moment counts so don't waste a second" and "Get Turbo Sleep." Even advice columnist Ann Landers added fuel to this fallacy. Near the top of her *Twenty-One Tips for Life* column, sleep ended up with some nasty bedfellows: "Don't believe all you hear, spend all you have, or sleep all you'd like." This implies that if you sleep all you like, you're probably a gullible, lazy spendthrift. Don't believe that!

Sleeping Less to Accomplish More

Our culture is rife with the notion that if you limit sleep, you can accomplish more. Many time-management experts advise adopting unhealthy sleep diets in the effort to get more done. In one very popular book about household organizing, the author charts a typical woman's day, allocating the hours of 4:30 to 6 A.M. and 10 to 11 P.M. for personal time and shaving sleep to an insufficient 5½ hours. Richard Carlson, in his best-seller *Don't Sweat the Small Stuff,* reveals that he gets up between 3 and 4 A.M. and recommends that readers consider a similar schedule.

Paradoxically, quality and efficiency diminish when sleep-deprived people try to squeeze it all in. The National Sleep Foundation states, "The body's need for sleep is treated as a waste of time. In our 24-hour society, we steal nighttime hours for daytime activities, cheating ourselves of precious sleep. In the past century, we have reduced our average sleep time by 20 percent, and in the past 25 years, added a month to our annual work/commute time. Our national sleep debt is on the rise. Our society has changed, but our bodies have not, and we are paying the price."

"The world might, indeed, be different if everyone got nine hours sleep, and if key decision makers were not among the least rested members of our society."

GAY GAER LUCE,
WRITER AND
RESEARCHER

4

Changing Habits That Hinder Sleep

Personal habits, some that have obvious effects and others that are more subtle, affect sleep quality. Daily routines, work, leisure activities, diet, sleeping partners, and travel can contribute to sleep problems. For instance, a calm career can help you relax, while a nightmarish work life can have the opposite effect.

The 7 Essential Habits of Highly Successful Sleepers

1. They give sleep top priority by assuring themselves ample sleep time.

2. They provide themselves with a comfortable place to sleep.

3. They choose daily activities that enhance their sleep.

4. They approach sleep problems as temporary challenges that can be remedied with creative perseverance.

5. They accommodate the physical changes and emotional transitions that negatively affect their sleep.

6. They replenish themselves with rest and relaxation.

7. They utilize outside resources to help assess and treat sleep problems.

How do you fare in comparison?

What you eat and drink during the day can enhance or inhibit your sleep potential. Also, think about what you do in the evening. Do you choose stimulating or sedating activities? Review your physical and emotional habits to learn which ones hinder sleep and to determine how to transform them into sleep enhancers.

Wake Up from Work Weariness

Does your job make you tired? Do you take work home with you, either in your overstuffed attaché case or in your overactive mind? Do you work many hours or have a long commute? Job stress affects sleep. One study found that workers who reported high levels of job stress had significantly more health problems than did those in less stressful jobs. Like insomnia, job burnout was correlated with an increase in allergies, migraines, backaches, and depression. Job stress and insomnia create a vicious cycle; more than two-thirds of adults report that sleepiness makes handling job stress even more difficult. Specific tasks can also affect sleep. For example, excessive computer work increases insomnia.

According to time-management consultant Donald Wetmore, M.B.A., J.D., 80 percent of employees do not want to go back to work on Monday morning. One long-term employee explains, "I generally don't have problems sleeping — except on Sundays. That's when I remember all the work that is piled on my desk from the week before and rerun in my head any client problems or staff arguments. I get up exhausted." If you are a reluctant Monday-morning worker, you are prone to the Sunday-night sleeping blues.

For many of us, the weekends just don't seem to be long enough to do all the chores and have enough time to relax and replenish our reserves. A *Shoe* comic strip illustrates this sentiment. Sitting up in bed, the character muses, "Morning again. Well, what did I expect; day follows night. But Monday should be cited for following too closely."

Why don't *you* wake up bright and cheery on Monday morning? Do you go to sleep late Sunday evening because you slept in

Sunday morning? Do you spend too much of your weekend doing chores, or do you take work home from the office? Your answers to these questions can guide you to design a better weekend-to-weekday transition.

Not surprisingly, working two jobs or having a long commute reduces sleep time and increases the risk of accidents. Researchers have found that workers with long commutes are more prone to sleep disorders. One study of 21,000 rail commuters points out that, in addition to cutting their sleep short to juggle their work schedules, commuters have higher levels of sleep apnea and insomnia. Another study found that drowsy drivers were twice as likely to be working more than one job and four to five times more likely to be working the night shift. Most dual-job workers averaged less than 6 hours of sleep. If working less is not an option, carpooling with more alert colleagues is a safer alternative.

Shift workers experience a greater incidence of insomnia, infertility, cardiovascular disorders, and other medical problems. These effects can be lessened with increased light while working at night and greater darkness during the day.

Shift workers can also benefit from changing the order of their routines. The average day worker's pattern is to follow work with leisure activities and, later, sleep. Those working nights should sleep after work and allocate the time between sleep and work for chores and recreation.

Human-resource professionals believe that additional sleep during the workday decreases stress and increases workers' efficiency. Trend forecasters list workplace napping as an important perk of the decade. Some businesses have already created corporate nap rooms at much less cost than fully equipped company exercise rooms. Dr. James Maas of Cornell University believes that "power naps," taken as short work breaks, may enhance an individual's job performance.

Would changing your job help you sleep better? The Buddhist concept of right livelihood encourages us to choose jobs that are aligned with our personal values and that contribute to the communal good. When we feel like victims of our jobs, we lose out emotionally, physically, and spiritually.

Drowsy Driving

The people most likely to drive while drowsy are those who are not getting enough sleep in the first place. These are the danger signs:

★ You have trouble focusing your eyes or keeping your head up.

★ You can't stop yawning.

★ You have wandering, disconnected thoughts.

★ You drift between lanes or have drifted off the road, and you keep jerking the car back into the lane.

If you experience any of these symptoms, pull your car over to a safe area and take a break or a nap. Start any trip by getting enough sleep the night before. Avoid driving during your body's downtime and take breaks during long trips.

Those who love their jobs often report refreshing sleep and renewed vigor when they return to their work tasks. If you don't look forward to your job, is it because you dislike your vocation or current situation? Think of your sleep or lack of it — especially on Sunday night — as a gauge of personal happiness. Only you can decide whether there is an underlying message.

Relaxing Refreshments

"You are what you eat." This popular slogan reflects the serious consequences our eating habits can have on our lives. Food affects health, vitality, and mood. When assessing a sleep problem, amend this phrase to "You sleep what you eat," since your choice of when and what you eat affects your sleep.

Schedule your evening meal at least 3 hours before bedtime. For better sleep, as well as overall health, eat a large breakfast, a moderate lunch, and a light dinner with a small portion of protein. Or eat smaller, more frequent meals throughout the day to maintain consistent blood sugar levels.

Ask yourself, "Does my daily diet promote health and sound sleep?" A heart-healthy, anticancer diet that is high in fiber, loaded with nutrient-rich fruits and veggies, and low in fat improves your general health and helps foster sleep.

Conversely, eating too many fatty foods can curtail your sleep. In *The Sleep Rx,* Norman Ford calls dietary fat a "gremlin food that promotes insomnia." Why the harsh characterization? Because, Ford explains, "Virtually every disease or dysfunction attributed to eating a high-fat diet and to being overweight has a detrimental effect on sleep and causes insomnia."

Vitamins and minerals are also important for sleep. "Nutritional deficiencies or poor absorption of nutrients can cause chronic insomnia," report Peter Hauri, Ph.D., and Shirley Linde, Ph.D., the authors of *No More Sleepless Nights.* Make sure to get your share of calming calcium.

The National Academy of Sciences' Institute of Medicine reports that the majority of Americans do not get sufficient amounts of calcium. Average consumption is 500 to 700 milligrams; most people need 1200 to 1500 milligrams. In addition to building strong bones and teeth, calcium helps regulate healthy nerve and muscle functioning. Supplemental calcium relieves premenstrual symptoms, too.

A combination of calcium and magnesium acts as a mild relaxant and sleep promoter. Other vitamins and minerals associated with sound sleep are the B vitamins, zinc, copper, and iron. A nutritionist can help you assess your need for supplementation.

Certainly, our overall nutritional status affects how we sleep, but can individual foods sedate or stimulate? Anecdotal accounts of sleep-inducing warm milk and turkey dinners seem to say so, yet the claims are not scientifically substantiated.

Many people believe that consuming foods with specific amino acids can help or hinder sleep. To induce sleep, turkey and other foods high in tryptophan have been recommended. Some experts counter that the legendary post–Thanksgiving dinner lethargy is really a result of overeating; the sedative effect of tryptophan occurs only if it is taken on an empty stomach with no protein present.

If you want to see whether tryptophan-laden foods have a sedative effect on you, try yogurt, turkey, peanut butter, dates, figs, rice, or tuna, all of which are high in tryptophan, an hour or so before bedtime. Avoid foods, including aged and soft cheeses, spinach, tomatoes, potatoes, and processed meats, that contain the energizing amino acid tyramine.

Nightcaps: Make Mine Milk

Will a glass of warm milk help you sleep? Scientists question the validity of this home remedy because the effects of milk's protein and stimulating amino acids may overpower the sedative effect of its tryptophan. But this calm culinary ritual, sweet childhood memories, and quiet time with your hands wrapped around a warm mug may also contribute to sound sleep.

Beware of other sleep-stealing foods. The additive monosodium glutamate (MSG) can cause headaches and insomnia in some folks. Check product labels for hydrolyzed protein, which contains MSG. Limit your intake of spicy, fatty, or fried foods, especially in the evening, as they can cause heartburn and indigestion. Energizing protein foods should be eaten earlier in the day; sugary snacks late in the day may be stimulating.

Carbohydrates, such as bread, cereal, and pasta, are good nighttime foods because they trigger the brain chemical serotonin, which makes you sleepy. Such a snack approximately 45 minutes before bed can sedate you. But keep it on the light side — a piece of toast with a little jam may do the trick.

Some health practitioners warn against eating refined carbohydrates at bedtime and suggest a small portion of fruit and almonds as an alternative evening snack. You may need to experiment with a few different snacks to find your best evening refreshment.

Jolting Substances

The major culprits of sound sleep are the jolting substances nicotine, alcohol, and caffeine. Several studies suggest that the stimulating effects of cigarette smoking steal sleep time. Heavy smokers tend to take longer to fall asleep, rouse more often, and experience less deep sleep. Some smokers wake up craving a cigarette during the night. In one study, those who quit their cigarette habits also cut their insomnia by half.

The paradox of alcohol is that it acts as both a relaxant and a stimulant. Some people insist that imbibing before bedtime helps them fall asleep. But physiological changes caused by alcohol deprive the body of needed rest. Drinking in the evening alters the natural sleep stages, making it harder to stay deeply asleep. It is also important to note that the process of withdrawing from nicotine and alcohol may initially increase insomnia in formerly heavy users.

Coffee drinkers, beware: Your habit may be hazardous to your sleep. The aroma of a freshly brewed cup of coffee and the jolt of alertness it brings make coffee drinking an attractive activity. But consuming 300 milligrams of caffeine, the equivalent of three cups of strong coffee or six cola drinks, at any time during a single day causes nighttime awakenings and disruption of the REM phase of sleep. Habitual coffee drinkers have excessively high levels of stress hormones and slightly elevated blood pressure many hours after coffee consumption.

Caffeine sensitivity increases with age. The snacks you once enjoyed, such as a cup of java in the afternoon or a slice of double chocolate cake for dessert, may now keep you up at night. Other stimulating substances that you may want to eliminate or reduce include chocolate, some over-the-counter medications, and coffee-flavored ice cream and yogurt.

If you are having sleep problems, you should bypass all beverages with a buzz. In addition to limiting coffee consumption, drink less tea and fewer soft drinks that have high caffeine levels. Tea drinking is charming and healthful, but it can be stimulating, too. The common green and black teas, which contain caffeine, give you a physiological boost and strong antioxidant protection. Tea's health benefits include reducing cancer risk, increasing cardiovascular strength, and normalizing intestinal flora. So savor your tea, but drink it 3 or more hours before bedtime.

Caffeine Counts

	AMOUNT CONSUMED	AMOUNT OF CAFFEINE
★ Coffee, brewed	8 oz.	80–135 mg.
★ Coffee, instant	8 oz.	65–100 mg.
★ Black tea	8 oz.	30–70 mg.
★ Green tea	8 oz.	25–50 mg.
★ Soda	12 oz.	30–70 mg.
★ Chocolate	1.5 oz.	5 mg.
★ Cold relief medicine	1 tablet	30 mg.

Don't Get Revved Up at Night

Do you have evening habits that stimulate you? A discussion of some of the most common routines that keep folks up at night may help you decide whether some of your activities need to be limited or eliminated, or whether a schedule change may help.

Often we are not aware of the effects of common habits. Many adults say that watching television relaxes them, and yet suspenseful and violent shows, including segments of the news, may be heart quickening. Late-night computer chats compete for our presleep attention and can also push us past a reasonable bedtime.

In her book *Gift from the Sea,* Anne Morrow Lindbergh describes the details of a visit with her sister at her beachside retreat. Lindbergh explains that after a day full of activity, "Evening is for sharing. Communication — but not for too long. Because good communication is as stimulating as black coffee, and just as hard to sleep after." Like Lindbergh, you may want to save your adrenaline-producing discussions for the daytime hours. Limit late-night phone calls, too, especially those concerning family tensions or work problems.

To ensure that exercise is sedating rather than stimulating, schedule it 3 hours or more before bedtime. Reschedule chores that may foster worry, such as paying bills, to a time earlier in the day. And don't save that exciting best-seller for bedtime — you may not be able to put it down or stop thinking about it once you do.

Break After-Hours Habits

Do you reluctantly abandon your comfortable bed at night because you have to go to the bathroom or eat a snack? These annoying practices can be remedied. Although it is important to keep hydrated during the day, limit your liquid intake within a few hours of bedtime. Coffee and alcohol cause many nighttime bathroom visits. Even if you are sipping sedative herbal tea, the portions should be controlled. Substituting a small dose of a medicinal liquid extract may lessen the need to urinate.

Some of us are conditioned to get up every time we wake up during the night. We automatically link awaking with urinating. Although it is recommended that you don't fight the urge to urinate during the night, experiment with not getting up immediately. People who are camping and don't have easy access to bathroom facilities often find that an extra evening trip is unnecessary. You may be able to recondition yourself at home, too.

Nocturia, or excessive urination at night, should be medically evaluated, since it may be a symptom of a urinary or vaginal infection or diabetes. Older men and pregnant women are most prone to extra nighttime bathroom trips. Most men over the age of 50 experience prostate enlargement, which causes increased frequency of urination. Prostate irritants include the usual culprits alcohol, caffeine, and tobacco, as well as spicy foods. Some self-help measures for prostate health include eating soy foods and pumpkin seeds and using the herb saw palmetto.

For pregnant women, hormonal changes and fetal growth increase pressure on the bladder, both day and night. Drinking less fluid close to bedtime may help. As body size increases, so does the inability to find comfortable sleeping positions. Cushioning the body with extra pillows, especially between the knees, and sleeping on the left side may lessen internal pressure and help curb nighttime urges to urinate.

What do you think of when you hear the term night eating? Many of us associate midnight snacks with the comic-strip character Dagwood Bumstead. But for others, night eating is a serious concern. It is a sleep-related eating disorder characterized by compulsive eating with possible purging and dissociative behaviors. If you make regular after-hours refrigerator raids, talk with a health-care professional.

Who Sleeps with You?

Do you share your bed? Do you sleep with another adult, with pets, or have an open family-bed policy? Do your evening sidekicks wake up often, have allergies, take up too much of the bed or the blankets, snore, watch late-night TV from bed, or go to sleep with cold feet? Do they have any habits that may be restricting your sleep? The sleep/ wake cycles of your bed partners can negatively affect you. Discussing the problem with them and making some physical changes may therefore be necessary.

Snoring affects approximately 30 to 40 percent of adults. For those who snore and their partners, the sound effects and health hazards are more than a noisy nuisance. Snoring can curb both intimacy and sleep. Sometimes separate bedrooms are necessary to assure the nonsnoring partner a good night's sleep. If your partner snores, recommend that he or she consult a health-care practitioner. There are remedies to lessen snoring. And snoring can be a symptom of sleep apnea, a disorder that requires medical treatment (see page 40).

One average-sized woman complained to her doctor of sleep problems. When queried, she revealed that she had recently remarried and her new husband, who was 6 feet tall and weighed 205 pounds, was now sharing her double bed. The problem sleeper had overlooked the obvious — that little mattresses are not good matches for big people. After purchasing a new king-size bed, the woman regained the deep sleep of her single years. Is your mattress large enough for you and your companion?

Another couple had to change sleeping positions to regain refreshing sleep. From the beginning of their 20-year relationship, they would fall asleep "spooning," their bodies in contact all night. This position was initially very comfortable for both partners and continued to be so until the woman approached menopause. "Now I don't like to be touched in bed at all when I am going to sleep. I've been having trouble with night sweats. My husband's body temperature irritates me."

After some discussion, the couple decided to sleep with a bit of distance between them. The recent change in their lives made them reevaluate a habit that had previously enhanced their sleep. There is an important lesson here: Are there any bed-sharing behaviors that no longer work for you?

"Oh, sleep it is a blessed thing, but not to those wakeful ones who watch their mates luxuriating in it when they feel that their own is sorely in arrears."

OGDEN NASH

Ease the Jet Lag Jitters

Whether you're flying to Europe to meet with an important business client or to begin a long-awaited vacation, if you don't watch out, there's a big chance that you'll feel . . . terrible. You may experience fatigue, disorientation, irritability, digestive disturbances, and problems sleeping after your arrival.

Jet lag is more than just being overtired from the physical demands of travel and excitement. It is a physiological disruption of the body's internal clock. Jet lag is caused by the need to adjust our sleep/wake cycle after crossing time zones. The National Aeronautics and Space Administration (NASA) estimates that a person needs one day for every time zone crossed to regain normal body rhythms and energy. For example, you cross five time zones when flying from New York to Paris; thus, it may take five days for your body to fully adjust.

No one is immune to jet lag; studies show that approximately 95 percent of long-distance travelers, including flight attendants, suffer from it.

Contributing Factors

There are a number of factors that contribute to the severity of jet lag. I've highlighted several of the most significant.

* Your direction of travel; jet lag tends to be worse when flying east than when flying west.
* Your age; the older you are, the worse jet lag is.
* Your preflight condition and degree of flexibility; you fare better if you are fit and rested and if you don't generally maintain a rigid schedule.
* Airline conditions; stale and dry cabin air and your lack of movement contribute to fatigue and lowered immunity.

Lessen the Effects of Jet Lag

Although you can't totally prevent jet lag, you can do some things to lessen its impact on your trip.

1. Preparation is key. Prior to your flight, make sure that you are well rested. Some experts suggest scheduling flights so that you don't leave very early in the morning but arrive in time for a full night's sleep.
2. Work to preset your biological clock. If you will be flying east, then the

week before you leave for your destination, start getting to bed earlier each day; if you will be flying west, stay up later and get up later.

3. During the flight, limit alcohol and drink plenty of water.

4. While on the plane, be sure to stretch your legs while in your seat, and try to walk around whenever possible.

5. Set your watch to the time at your destination and eat and sleep according to the new schedule (this may mean refusing some of the airline meals — which many may say is not a loss!).

6. Try using eyeshades and earplugs to sleep better on the plane.

7. Some folks take an antihistamine for its sleep-inducing properties, but this medicine can also cause negative side effects, including dehydration.

8. When you arrive, continue to follow your new pattern. Try not to nap.

9. Sunlight and mild exercise early in the day help reset your body's clock as quickly as possible.

10. It also makes sense to use scents to adjust to time shifts. Purchase or make aromatherapy products specifically for use during and after your flight. You can bring a sleep pillow with you or a small bottle of your favorite calming scent (see pages 158–160 for more information and recipes).

11. Supplemental melatonin, taken 30 minutes before your new bedtime, can help lessen jet lag and reset your body's clock (see page 166).

"A well-spent day brings happy sleep"

LEONARDO DA VINCI

5

Dream Up a Sleep-Inviting Environment

A calm home provides a respite after full and often frenetic days spent out in the world. When we walk in our front doors and are greeted by blaring stereos, glaring lights, loud colors, and bold patterns, our senses stay on overdrive.

Of course, we all need areas in our homes for stimulating activities. But for balance, we also need peaceful spaces that soothe our senses and signal us to switch from activity to quiet. Innovative decorating, comfortable bedding, and correct lighting can help you transform your bedroom into a sleep-inviting environment.

A Soothing Sleep Setting

"The feather pillow and the quilt are to repose what champagne and chocolate mousse are to diet."

LYNNE SHARON SCHWARTZ, NOVELIST

Is your bedroom conducive to sound sleep? Your sleep space should be calm, comfortable, clean, and cozy. While mental clutter may keep you from falling asleep, physical clutter in the bedroom, such as piles of dirty clothes, unwieldy stacks of magazines, or too many knickknacks, can also distract. Spend some time cleaning out the mess.

In addition, don't allow your bedroom to do double duty as a mini office. Put the desk and the computer in another room or screen them from view. Relocate the television and answering machine. If you keep a telephone by the bed to increase your sense of safety and security, turn the ringer to low. Reserve your bedroom for only three things — sleeping, reflecting, and romancing.

According to the principles of feng shui, the ancient Oriental art of object placement, positioning your bed correctly can improve your sleep as well as your relationships. For optimum health, never put your bed in a direct line with a door or a bathroom. Don't place your bed under beams and don't store items under your bed.

To transform your bedroom into a restful sanctuary, eliminate flashy or distracting artwork, bedding, wall coverings, and window treatments. For serene surroundings, add gently flowing fabrics and soft music. Decorate with light blues and greens. View only gentle beauty from your bed to enhance your moods and the quality of your sleep.

Make your bedroom a relaxation haven by paging through magazines, cutting out some pictures, and creating a file of serene bedroom scenes. What do you like about these rooms? Find the similarities in colors, shapes, and textures. Choose three things you could change in your bedroom that would make it more relaxing.

Bed-and-breakfast inns can provide inspiration. Their proprietors often entice us with theme-oriented rooms and special treats. Have you ever stayed in, or wanted to stay in, the Garden Room, the Emily Dickinson Room, or the Blue Room? Copy B&B-style amenities and small indulgences in your own home, such as a decorating scheme, soft colors, fresh flowers, a canopied bed, or a comfy chaise longue. The most important thing is to learn to associate sleep and calm with your restful bedroom.

A Cool, Quiet Bedroom

Is your bedroom cool enough? Turn down the heat to save on fuel bills while you create an ideal sleeping environment. Reset your thermostat to the recommended sleeping temperature of 65°F (18°C). Should you sleep with the windows open or closed? Obviously, it depends on your comfort level and where you live. Safety factors, noise, and drafts should be considered. But stuffy rooms can impede deep sleep, and opening the window a crack can help. After a week has passed, decide whether the new temperature is right for you.

Warm Feet for Deep Sleep

To enhance sleep during the winter months, be sure to supplement your cool room with warm socks or a hot-water bottle. Warm feet are a natural sedative. Studies show that they help you fall asleep better than calming foods and supplements.

In addition, shield yourself from noises you cannot control, such as street sounds and airplane noise, and from those you can, including loud stereos and television sets. Mask unpleasant noises with consistent low-level background sound from a "white-noise" machine or a fan. Many people find that the constant hum lulls them to sleep.

Try other soundproofing strategies, such as installing wall hangings and rugs to insulate against noise from adjoining rooms or apartments. Heavy curtains muffle outside noise. Earplugs may be another defense. College students often benefit from the policy of dormitory "quiet hours" after 10 P.M. What kind of policy can you adopt at your house?

Many bedrooms are too dry, especially in the winter. If you suffer from nosebleeds or a sore or dry throat, a lack of moisture may be the cause. Consider buying a humidifier. Check the manufacturer's instructions; if possible, add a few drops of lavender, chamomile, or another fragrant, sedative essential oil.

Allergies also contribute to poor sleep. Wash your bedding regularly in hot water to get rid of dust mites. Consult an allergist or a health-care professional about purchasing air filters and using the latest methods to reduce mites, molds, and other airborne allergens in your bedroom.

Sleep Enhancers

Anthropologists remind us that people in many cultures have successfully slept on the ground and on skins, mats, and wooden platforms. Pillows and head supports were once rare; extrafirm mattresses, box springs, and futons are modern-day inventions. Thankfully, they enhance the bedtime experience, as do sensuous sheets and fluffy pillows. Other practical and aesthetic details can transform the space where you sleep into your own cradle of comfort.

First, assess your bed. Is it old and lumpy? Does it sag? If so, replace your mattress. The trend is toward larger beds and thicker mattresses. Mattress choices include innerspring and box spring combinations, foam pads, futons, air beds, and water beds.

These choices are subjective. *The University of California, Berkeley, Wellness Letter* explains, "The idea that there is a 'best' bed exists mostly in ad copy. There is no scientific consensus on what makes a good mattress." For practical advice about mattress shopping, check *Consumer Reports.*

After a long, stressful day, ensure yourself a foundation of rest. Sink into the caresses of a feather bed. Indulge in comfortable covers and a plush comforter. Down is a good choice for bedcovers, but

"Always buy a good bed and a good pair of shoes. If you're not in one, you're in the other."

GLORIA HUNNIFORD,
BRITISH TALK-SHOW
HOST

synthetic alternatives launder more easily and reduce allergic reactions. Versatile duvet covers, which are essentially pillow-cases for your comforter, let you update fabrics for decorative purposes and seasonal weight and are easy to wash.

Buy the softest sheets you can afford. In a recent survey of 500 American women, 93 percent said they believe that quality sheets result in a better night's sleep. Some swear by silk or satin. Choose all-cotton sheets to keep you cool in the summer and try a set of fuzzy flannel ones to warm you up in the winter. Also, consider a sheet's thread count, the number of woven threads used per square inch. Higher thread counts denote higher quality, durability, and cost. Sheets with 200 or more threads per square inch also feel softer.

Purchase a new pillow. Feather and down pillows are pricey but comfortable and, gen-erally, last longer than their synthetic counterparts. Choose one based on support and comfort. A pillow's capacity to keep your neck and spine in proper alignment is related to your sleeping position. Side sleepers benefit from a firm foam pillow. An additional pillow between your legs helps reduce pressure on the lower back and hips. Back sleepers are better off with a flatter pillow or one filled with soft down. Avoid sleeping on your stomach, if possible, since this practice puts the most strain on your back.

Don't neglect to replace your "broken" pillows. Test one by folding it in half; if the pillow stays folded and does not return to its original position, it's time to purchase a new one.

Let There Be Light

The discovery of the lightbulb changed our society from one that revolved around limited daylight hours to our present 24-hour lifestyle. Electricity made it possible for us to get up before the sun, work all shifts, and prolong evening activities as long as desired. But artificial light contributes to the decrease in the average number of hours we sleep and throws our natural cycles out of sync.

Bedroom lighting should be soft, not bright. Some people are especially sensitive to light when they are trying to fall asleep. Turn off the television and cover a bright clock. If glaring streetlights keep you awake, use dark window curtains or eye-shades to screen them out.

When you get up to use the bathroom during the night, or wake up with a dream and want to write it down, keep the lights low. Bright bulbs can trick your body into thinking it is morning and time to get up. Use dimmer switches and night-lights in dark hallways and bathrooms. Purchase a small flashlight or special penlight for middle-of-the-night jottings.

If you are sleep challenged, take a walk in natural daylight early in the day. Bright light in the morning and subdued light at night help keep our bodies attuned to their natural rhythms. Alarm clocks with special lights, called dawn simulators, replicate the gradual rising of the morning sun and may help you greet the day more readily.

Seasonal Affective Disorder

Do you sleep more in the winter but feel less rested? Gray and gloomy weather may affect your mood as well as your sleep habits. Waning winter light appears to cause seasonal affective disorder (SAD), which is estimated to affect more than 10 million American adults.

The effects of SAD have been likened to those of a continuous case of jet lag. SAD sufferers are prone to awake in the morning feeling as though it were still the middle of the night. Other symptoms of this physiologically based form of clinical depression include lethargy, eating more and excessive cravings for carbohydrates, weight gain, feeling blue, and sleeping more than usual.

Light therapy appears to help sufferers. Experts recommend taking early-morning walks outdoors and using a commercial light box or lighted visor while indoors.

6

Self-Help Strategies

Don't be a victim of your sleeplessness! Too many people endure the frustration and fatigue of sleepless nights, resigning themselves to what they consider to be their inevitable fate. Although you have no conscious control over sleep, you can change your circumstances to encourage better slumber.

Try empowering self-help strategies, such as soothing rituals, relaxing baths, behavior modification, naps, exercise, and inspiration from others, to alter your attitudes about sleep and reduce your sleep-robbing anxieties. Utilizing these techniques will increase your chances of transforming long sleepless nights into more restful ones.

Bedtime Rituals

"What a fine night for sleeping! From all that I hear, It's the best night for sleeping in many a year."

Parents often create soothing bedtime rituals for their children. A bath, followed by some cuddling in a rocking chair and a lullaby or a story read aloud, gives the evening an expected structure that helps little ones slowly release the day. Adults also need soothing ways to switch from busyness to slower, quieter evenings.

Bedtime rituals are especially helpful for those who live hectic lives full of decision making and crises. Not much thought is required when you have designed a restful routine, as the pre-established rhythm creates a pleasant cycle of expectation.

Sleep Guidelines

★ Establish a sleep schedule: Go to sleep at the same time every night and wake up at the same time every morning. When this is not possible, remember that a regular evening curfew is helpful but keeping a consistent waking time is even more important.

★ Allow yourself enough sleep time. Nap when needed.

★ If you do need to catch up on your sleep over the weekend, extend your sleep time by only an hour or two.

★ Create bedtime rituals that slow you down and help your transition to sleep.

★ Don't try too hard to sleep; it won't work. When sleep researchers offered study volunteers $25 if they could fall asleep quickly, subjects took twice as long to fall asleep as the volunteers who didn't have this enticement — and the pressure.

Bedtime Traditions

Choose from these ideas to create your own bedtime ritual:

- ★ Take a warm herbal bath.
- ★ Soak in a sauna, whirlpool, or hot tub.
- ★ Close the bedroom door for quiet time.
- ★ Relax in a comfortable chair.
- ★ Listen to soft instrumental music.
- ★ Peruse the pages of a magazine.
- ★ Reflect on some inspirational readings.
- ★ Write in a journal or pen a personal note.
- ★ Call a good friend.
- ★ Savor a cup of herbal tea.
- ★ Do some gentle stretching exercises.
- ★ Pray.
- ★ Breathe deeply.
- ★ Sing a song.
- ★ Look at photos of a relaxing vacation.
- ★ Knit, crochet, or quilt.
- ★ Gaze at the stars.
- ★ Imagine yourself contentedly sleeping.

Will you need any supplies? Perhaps you'll want to purchase some bath salts, a blank book for journal entries, a new novel or CD.

To design your own bedtime ritual, choose one to three new ways to wind down. Try these activities for seven nights. At the end of the week, ask yourself if you were more relaxed in the evening, if it was any easier to fall asleep, and if your overall sleep comfort improved. Add or change activities on the basis of your honest evaluation. Remember that it takes three weeks to create a new habit and three months for the habit to become second nature.

Evening Anxieties

Best-selling author Wally Lamb describes his evening worrying in a breathless phrase. While he was feeling the pressure about his not-yet-written second novel, he says he had "a terrible time at first. A frightening, wake-up-at-2-A.M.-and-stay-up-for-the-rest-of-the-night-with-a-fist-in-the-gut kind of time of it."

How many of us have experienced nights like that? The unfinished business that keeps us stressed during the day and wide awake at night may include practical work details,

"She cannot tell which disturbs her sleep more, the future or the past."

ALICE HOFFMAN, NOVELIST

home projects, or leftover emotions, such as anger or fear. Just as we lay our head on the pillow, our internal sportscaster may begin a replay of the day's fumbles as well as its touchdowns. Here are some techniques that can help lessen the time and energy we expend on these mental gymnastics.

K. Albert, M.D., Ph.D., former director of a New York City sleep laboratory, states in her book *Get a Good Night's Sleep,* "Your sleeping life and your waking life are one." To treat sleep problems effectively, we must first figure out how one life affects the other.

Dr. Albert suggests that a direct, logical approach may not always work and that a different perspective, one that calls on our intuitive and playful side, may provide helpful answers. She suggests completing revealing statements such as these:

1. If I could make one wish about my sleep, it would be _____.
2. The last time I fell asleep easily was _____.
3. I know exactly what I need to do to regain my sleep, and that is _____.

Your spontaneous responses can give you clues to the cause of your sleep problems and point you in the direction of creative solutions.

It may also help to write in a journal. Researchers have found that journal writing benefits emotional and physical health. Regular entries will help you express your thoughts and feelings, many of which, when unacknowledged, impede your sleep. One longtime diarist explains, "During stressful times, when anxiety is keeping me awake at night, emptying my worries onto paper calms me down and lets me get a good night's sleep."

Some people find that when they keep a to-do list, they ruminate less before sleep and don't awake as often fretting about a forgotten task. At the end of your workday or before dinner, take 5 or 10 minutes to review the day's accomplishments and any activities left undone. Compile a list of things that you plan to do the next day and rank them in order of importance. A notebook and pen on your bedside table can catch any late-night reminders.

"Fun is something grown-ups never have before bedtime, only after."

JUDITH VIORST,
POET AND
JOURNALIST

Insomnia can become a self-fulfilling prophecy. The cycle of fear is punctuated by frantic questions such as "What if I can't sleep again tonight? I just can't miss any more sleep." If this sounds familiar, have faith; you will sleep again.

Talking with a friend can help you regain your perspective. Pressure to sleep exacerbates the problem. Alleviate some of the stress by allowing yourself alternatives, such as an occasional late wake-up time, or a day off after a sleepless night.

If you think that your insomnia is related to depression or anxiety, consult a mental-health professional who can help you figure out the cause of your sleep problems and choose strategies to solve them. In one study, more than 75 percent of chronic insomniacs who received psychotherapy benefited from the experience.

Exercise to Sleep Easy

One of the wonderful health-promoting benefits of exercise is that it can help keep you awake during the day and improve your sleep at night. More than 70 percent of people say that they don't work out because they are too tired; but what they may not know is that exercise is a great stress reliever. When you break the fatigue/inactivity cycle, you're energized by the movement and rewarded with subsequent relaxation.

In one study, adults who engaged in moderate exercise four times a week for 30 to 40 minutes had greater improvement in their sleep than did their sedentary counterparts. The exercisers slept nearly an hour longer at night, took less time to fall asleep, and took fewer daytime naps. Another poll found that those who walked at least six blocks a day at a normal pace were one-third less likely to have trouble staying asleep than were non-walkers. People who walked a bit more briskly actually slashed their risk of a sleep disorder by 50 percent!

Daily exercise also helps lessen the risks of a wide range of problems, from heart disease to depression and insomnia. Inactivity is linked to at least 15 chronic diseases. Thirty minutes of moderate daily exercise is recommended.

Weight-bearing exercise keeps us strong and flexible and wards off osteoporosis. If muscle or joint aches keep you awake, try smooth stretching movements to ease stiffness and pain. Yoga, tai chi, and calisthenics involve movements that increase flexibility.

Make an exercise appointment with yourself. Go jogging, ride a bicycle, swim, or work in the garden. Scheduling an aerobics class at a gym or community center can motivate you to stick with it. It's even better if you sign up with a friend. Whatever you do, consistency is the key.

Timing your exercise sessions is also important. Early-morning exercisers are often pleased to have accomplished the task prior to the required activities of the day, but, in general, early exercise doesn't affect evening sleep. In fact, those who exercise at the beginning of the day, especially if they get up extra early to fit it in, seem to reach their energy peak by the afternoon and get tired after lunch.

Afternoon workouts seem to have the most benefit for those with sleeping problems. They help increase afternoon alertness and deepen evening sleep. However, do not exercise within three hours of bedtime. This time cushion will allow your body to slow down and its temperature to readjust.

Go to Bed when Sleepy

Go to bed when you're sleepy. Many people go to bed when they think they should, rather than when they are tired. Although this advice seems to contradict the sleep hygiene tip about sticking to a curfew, if you suffer from insomnia, you may need to experiment to determine your best sleep time. As you approach your designated bedtime, ask yourself, "Am I tired? How many hours did I sleep last night? How active have I been today? Am I ready for sleep?"

If you can't sleep, get up. Often insomnia is a sign that we are out of sync with our cycles and habits. If you experience insomnia, you may need to relearn healthful bedtime practices.

Richard Bootzin, Ph.D., a sleep expert, developed a behavioral technique that stresses the important association between your bed and falling asleep quickly and easily. Dr. Bootzin recommends that if you haven't fallen asleep within 10 minutes of getting into bed, you should get up. Cut out all afternoon naps and curb reading and watching television in bed. If you wake up during the night and can't go back to sleep within 10 minutes, the same rule applies: Get up. Get back into bed only when you feel tired.

Initially, an insomniac may get up a number of times during the night. But if insomnia is caused by a disturbed sleep habit, this technique can help substitute a new and better sleep routine. Studies show a marked improvement in sleep after consistent use of this technique over a two-week period.

Other sleep experts emphasize the reparative aspects of rest. Deepak Chopra, M.D., disagrees with suggestions for getting up and occupying yourself when you are not sleeping. He believes that even if you can't sleep, you will benefit from relaxation.

In his book *Restful Sleep*, Chopra recommends that once you get into bed, you should "assume a comfortable position and don't worry about sleeping. Let your mind wander freely. Take the attitude that you will get as much rest as nature wants you to have at that moment, as much as you need, even if you're not actually sleeping. Sleep will come naturally when it comes, and meanwhile you're gaining the benefit of valuable rest and rejuvenation of your whole system."

Revitalize with a Nap

Naps are fabulous fatigue fighters. With no equipment to purchase or techniques to learn, naps help us relax and remedy daytime sleepiness. Think of NAPS as *Natural Afternoon Pleasure Sleep* and grab your blanket and a pillow to doze off anywhere. And for those who feel guilty and fear losing their job or their reputation, consider NAPS *Normal Afternoon Productivity Sleep.*

Critics of napping liken it to snacking and admonish that both can ruin your appetite for the "real meal." In a survey of committed nappers, those who dozed during the day complained that they got dirty looks from

"Never make a major decision until after you've taken a nap."

SARAH BAN
BREATHNACH,
AUTHOR

their parents, roommates, or spouses and were accused of being lazy.

Nappers often feel guilty about their seeming indulgence. But daytime sleep breaks can lessen your sleep debt and allow you to be more efficient and creative. A quick snooze provides healthy relief from stress.

Studies by university researchers show that "prophylactic napping," or napping in advance of a long stretch of activity, can improve one's memory, mood, judgment, and creativity. Naps may also decrease accidents, both on and off the road. All that from a little shut-eye!

How do naps affect nighttime sleep? Timing is everything. The lull between 2 and 4 P.M., signaled by a natural dip in our body temperature, is a favorite time to slow down and curl up. Just don't nap later in the day. If you do, it may be more difficult to fall asleep at night. The best naps last from 20 minutes to an hour. Longer than that and there is a good chance that you will wake up feeling groggy rather than refreshed.

Where should you nap? Don't waste your precious nap time falling asleep in front of the TV. Get comfy. At home, the bed and the couch are in close running for favorite nap spot. People list a variety of strange places where they nap when on the go — in their car, in a library cubicle, or in a bathroom stall! About one out of six adults report that their employers allow them to take naps at work.

Notable Nappers

Many presidents and other politicians, actors and artists, and other movers and shakers have something in common — they nap(ped). Join the list of famous siesta snoozers, including John F. Kennedy, Jr., Winston Churchill, Sophia Loren, Leonardo da Vinci, Albert Einstein, and Rip van Winkle.

Do you have a favorite season to nap? Picture a winter weekend, coming indoors after skiing or shoveling snow, a warm bowl of soup for lunch, followed by an afternoon nap. Or a summer vacation nap, on the beach or at the hotel, as the perfect segue between daytime sight-seeing and a light evening meal. Visualize your perfect nap place and time.

Soothe in a Sedative Soak

Water naturally calms our senses. Whether listening to the soothing sound of the surf, sitting by the water's edge, swimming, soaking in a hydrotherapy spa treatment, or luxuriating in the comfort of your own bathtub, you'll find water relaxing.

Physiologically, baths help promote rest, since there is a correlation between body temperature and sleep. Our body temperature has a normal fluctuation of about 1½ to 2 degrees, with a peak in the late morning or early afternoon and a decline in the evening. We get sleepy when our body temperatures naturally drop in the evening. That drop is assisted when we cool off after a bath.

Close the bathroom door and shut out the world. Fill the bath with warm water. Dim the lights or use candles to gently illuminate the space. Try an eye mask or compress to soothe tired eyes and tense temple muscles. Recline with a waterproof neck pillow or place a rolled-up towel behind your neck. Play some soft instrumental music. Slip into solitude and let the day go. This ritual provides a gentle invitation to sleep.

You can also slow down with a shower. Showers are mistakenly viewed as the stimulating sibling of the more sedating bath. But steamy showers can be sensuous and relaxing. Linger and let the water massage your tight muscles.

To double the benefits of bathing, try a relaxing Epsom salts bath and shower combo. After a tiring day, loosen taut muscles in a tub filled with two cups of Epsom salts and hot water (stimulating but not scalding!). Sink into the bath, and lounge with a towel or bath pillow behind your head. When the bathwater begins to cool, stand up and turn on the shower. Rinse yourself off with a blast of cold water, then end with a warming stream.

Pace, Plan, and Prepare

As Simon and Garfunkel sang, "Slow down, you move too fast." The accelerated pace of contemporary life, marked by increasing responsibilities and activities, leaves little time to rest and replenish our reserves.

Pace Yourself

We treat ourselves mechanistically, acting as if we could turn on and off as easily as a light switch. We expect to go directly from high gear to sleep, then wake up the next morning alert and ready to spring into action. However, we need time to move from one phase to another.

Imagine an ideal evening or a perfect morning. What time would you go to sleep and wake up to allow for sufficient sleep? Would you set aside some time to stretch or exercise? Write in your journal or say prayers? How would you greet the new day and how would you let it end? Design graceful bedtimes and awakenings by incorporating some of your ideas into your schedule this week.

Plan Ahead

It's often difficult to sleep the night before a big event. Just when a good night's sleep is needed to fortify us for the demands of a job interview or the pleasures of a vacation, our anxiety can keep us awake. One solution is not to cram. Allocate extra time for mental and physical preparation. Pack your suitcase or review your notes earlier in the day. Then use the time right before bed for a bath, massage, or other form of relaxation.

Approach Tomorrow Prepared

Do you pleasantly anticipate tomorrow or anxiously dread it? How you feel about the next day's activities can affect your sleep. Let's face it, mornings in most households are chaotic. There's the chorus of alarm clocks, arguments about whose turn it is for the bathroom, the search for lost shoes, breakfasts to serve, lunches to make, and inspections to ensure that everyone has the right backpack, then wondering, as you walk out the door, "Did I feed the dog?" Many people choose to solve the problem of hectic mornings by waking up very early or

"Often I'll find that if I go to sleep laying the day's problems out to myself, I'll more or less consistently wake up with a solution."

ART SPIEGELMAN,
WRITER AND
CARTOONIST

stretching the evening, spending the precious before bedtime hour trying to get it all done. What else can you do?

An effective long-term approach incorporates planning, preparation, and shared responsibilities. Designate a family prep time. Take 30 minutes in the early evening to prepare for the next day's activities. While you're cooking dinner, have the kids pack their school sack or pick out the next day's clothes. Design, delegate, and delete — outline what needs to be done, eliminate what you can, and get to bed on time.

How Others Cope

Knowing you're not the only one watching late-night TV or scribing e-mails in the wee morning hours may be somewhat comforting, but it doesn't help you catch the Zs you need to feel refreshed tomorrow. How do others cope with sleeplessness? I asked a number of people what they do. Following are a collection of the answers I received.

"I calm down by calling a good friend who works on second shift. If I can't sleep, around midnight we'll get on the phone for half an hour or so and it helps both of us get settled in."

"I go outside. Even if it's late and cold. A few minutes of breathing the fresh air and looking at the stars helps me get back to bed."

"My mother used to make me warm milk at night. It still seems to work; maybe it's the minerals, or being in the kitchen, or maybe it's just the memories. But it helps me get to sleep."

"Have you read *Simple Abundance?* The author suggests keeping a 'gratitude journal.' Now when I can't sleep, I get up and write down five things that happened that day, big or small, that I'm grateful for. It always puts things in perspective and I stop worrying about the bad things long enough to fall asleep."

"Reading puts me to sleep. Books, magazines, as long as they're not too suspenseful or sad. Reading in bed is often the first time I've stopped moving all day. I really enjoy a quiet 15 minutes, and then I fall asleep easily."

"I put on a new CD and lie down with a warm compress on my head. And drift off."

"When I can't sleep, my partner gives me a massage. Mmmm . . . rubs my back and feet, and by then I'm out."

"I sit down and play a tune on the piano. Not a new one I'm trying to learn but an old, easy favorite. It's soothing to perform."

"I play the day backward in my head. I used to worry about how much I hadn't got done. Now I'm surprised at how much I've actually accomplished. I feel more peaceful, and then I can fall asleep."

"How do people go to sleep? I'm afraid I've lost the knack."

DOROTHY PARKER,
POET AND HUMORIST

"When I've been having trouble sleeping for a few days, I decide to keep really busy the next day. I just exhaust myself, and then at bedtime I fall asleep quickly, almost when I put my head on the pillow."

"Being outdoors and being active during the day help me sleep at night. Seasonal activities — like gardening and swimming or skiing and wood splitting. I think that both the exertion and the keeping in touch with nature help."

7

Relax, You Are Getting Sleepy...

Do you lie awake worrying about the bills, the children, your health, or what the boss said yesterday? While in bed, do you plan the itinerary for your upcoming vacation or outline the next Great American Novel? Your own thoughts may be the biggest obstacle to your getting a refreshing night's sleep.

If your ideas and anxieties are impeding your sleep, there are a number of methods you can use to calm your overactive mind while soothing your tense body. Learn to use two of your natural allies, your breath and your imagination, to surrender to sleep. Relaxation techniques, including progressive muscle relaxation, yoga, music therapy, meditation, massage, and bodywork, can also increase your ability to sleep deeply.

Lessen Stress

According to a recent study, people who practiced stress reduction techniques while weaning themselves off sleeping pills slept better and had fewer withdrawal symptoms than those who didn't use stress management methods. Research has also shown that people who combine relaxation techniques with other natural sleep-inducing methods experience deeper and more refreshing sleep.

Take a Deep Breath

Learn to breathe? What's to learn? Isn't it a natural process? Yes, but . . .

Stress, poor posture, and our cultural obsession with tight abs are some obstacles to deep breathing. For optimal health, breathing should be full and rhythmic, using the diaphragm and ribs to fill and empty the lungs. When you take a full, diaphragmatic breath, there is a gentle flow of air in and out of your nostrils. As you inhale, your stomach and chest expand and rise; as you exhale, they contract. There should be little, if any, noise.

"If I had to limit my advice on healthier living to just one tip, it would be simply to learn how to breathe correctly."

ANDREW WEIL, M.D.

You can alleviate end-of-the-day anxiety by consciously altering the rhythm and depth of your breathing. The relaxation that results from deep breathing can help you let go and let sleep come. To discharge stress and prepare for bed, take a couple of cleansing breaths. Take a deep breath in through your nose, and then let it out audibly through puckered lips, as though you were blowing out a candle. Repeat.

Breathe Yourself to Sleep

Janet Wilson, who has taught yoga for more than 25 years, recommends this breathing technique for people who have sleep problems. It combines two important elements of relaxation: deep breathing and mental focus.

1. Lie on your back in bed. Take 4 diaphragmatic breaths (long, slow, and deep) through your nose.

2. Turn onto your left side and take 8 diaphragmatic breaths.

3. Return to your back and take 16 breaths.

4. Then (if you are still awake), turn onto your right side and take 32 breaths.

5. Continue to turn in this sequence, doubling the number of breaths with each turn.

Janet reassures me that people usually fall asleep long before they have exhausted their mathematical skills.

Lengthening your exhalation, then holding after all the air is expelled, is also very relaxing. To benefit from some slow, calming breaths, inhale to a silent count of four, hold for a count of one, quietly exhale to a count of eight, and then hold for a count of four. Imagine breathing in quiet and stillness and breathing out noise and tension.

Another technique is to lie in bed comfortably on your back. Shift your awareness to your breath. Simply paying attention to your breathing without trying to change it can begin to calm you. After a couple of minutes, put one hand on your chest and the other on your abdomen. Create a quiet wave between your chest and belly by slowing and deepening your breath. You can also alter your breathing while listening to slow instrumental music.

Visualization Exercises

Play some peaceful "mind movies" before bed. When you visualize, you use your imagination as a sleep-enhancing ally. Visualizing tranquil images engages your calm and creative center, and focusing on a repetitive image leaves little brain space for the worries that keep you awake.

As the director of a focused and relaxed internal reverie, you can imagine a scene with all of your senses. For example, when I hear the lyrics "Picture yourself on a boat on a river with tangerine trees and marmalade skies," I not only envision a soothing place, but also imagine the light wind on my skin (how it feels) and a mild, sweet aroma (how it smells).

Want to try visualization to relax yourself to sleep? Inspiration for calm scenes can come from personal experience (remember that secluded beach you once visited?) or can be found on picture postcards or in nature-oriented magazines. What does your peaceful place look like, feel like, smell like? Is it warm and sunny, or cool and invigorating? Do not include other people in the image; the place is yours alone. Here are some images to inspire you to create your own "mind movies":

★ Count sheep. This old standby still has merit. Imagining leaping lambs as you lie down is a simple way to relax with a calm image and an uncomplicated mental focus.

★ Subtract stress. Studies show that when people count backward, they experience positive and relaxing physiological changes. You can count yourself to calm by picturing a simple scoreboard slowly shifting from the numbers 100 to 0. If this method is not strong enough to soothe you, try to subtract some of your worry time with another math challenge. Imagine numbered signs with your answers as you silently count backward from 100 in groups of seven.

★ Picture serene nature scenes. After lights-out, take a few deep, cleansing breaths, and then paint a mind picture of a quiet place. Imagine a peaceful lakeshore. See the water's sparkling ripples, feel the gentle breeze, hear the call of the loons, and smell the fresh air. Picture yourself sitting there alone, breathing slowly and enjoying the tranquillity of the outdoors.

★ Imagine yourself in a field of wild-flowers. Picture a Monet canvas of a field of poppies. Walk across the vibrant meadow with the sun shimmering behind you. Stay as long as you want to in this safe spot.

Guided Imagery

Guided imagery, a more directed visualization method, has proved to be a powerful tool for health and healing. You can listen to a scripted audiotape, or a counselor can help you design an individualized image.

The Academy for Guided Imagery reports, "A growing body of medical research shows that imagery has a powerful influence on every major control system of the body, stimulating vital functions like heart rate, blood pressure, local blood flow, wound healing, and even immune functioning." Many of these changes foster relaxation and enhance sleep.

★ Visualize a way to release your worries. Lie quietly with your eyes closed. Picture a basket on your lap. Name your burdensome concerns, one by one, as you put them into the container. Imagine walking to a stream and pouring the basket's contents into the water. Watch your worries float away.

Progressive Muscle Relaxation

Progressive muscle relaxation (PMR) is a wonderfully simple but powerful technique that involves tensing and releasing different muscle groups in a specific sequence. The technique works because muscle relaxation and anxiety are incompatible. As you contract and release your muscles, you will experience an accompanying release of stress. I know a man who was experiencing insomnia and learned PMR in a yoga class. His wife reports that whenever he has trouble sleeping, he does PMR in bed, "and then he's out like a light." It can work for you, too.

How to Do PMR

1. Find a comfortable position. During the day, you may want to practice in a chair. At bedtime, lie on your back in bed. Take a few minutes to squirm around until it feels like your body fits the bed.

2. Beginning with your feet and progressing up your body, tense and then relax each muscle group. First, tighten your left foot, pointing your toes and stretching as far as it is comfortable. Don't strain. The initial tendency is to hold your breath when you tighten; instead, consciously continue to breathe slowly and fully. Hold the position for five seconds. Then release your foot.

3. It is easier to experience the true relaxation of a muscle when you compare it with the feel of a tight one. Do you notice any difference between your left foot and your right one? You may sense a lightness, heaviness, lengthening, looseness, or warmth in your left foot. These are some of the

"Tired nature's sweet restorer, balmy sleep!"

EDWARD YOUNG

ways people describe the feelings of muscle relaxation.

4. Do the same tightening and releasing of your right foot. Then move up to your calf, knee, and thigh muscles. Continue to be aware of your breathing. Alternate tightening and releasing the right and left sides of your body. Tense the muscle, hold, and release.

5. Move up to the groin, buttocks, and stomach area, followed by your back, arms, and hands.

6. Proceed to tighten and release your neck, face, and head. Scrunch your jaw muscles, and then release. Squeeze your eyes shut, hold, and then release. Proceed to your forehead.

7. End by rubbing your hands together and gently placing your palms over your eyes.

Masterful Meditation

Meditation is the premier method for calming the constant stream of thoughts and images in our overactive brains. It also helps us experience relaxation and a sense of living in the present moment. Those who meditate regularly claim that the practice is a powerful tool to enhance overall physical health, emotional well-being, and spiritual serenity.

Meditation can be practiced at any time of day or night. You may feel some benefits immediately after a meditation session, but, as with other relaxation techniques, the positive effects are cumulative.

For best results, establish a consistent time and place to meditate. The evening is a good time for stillness and reflection, and meditation can help you slow down for the transition to sleep. Those who awake in the middle of the night bothered by too many thoughts to easily fall back to sleep find that a minimeditation in bed often helps clear their mind.

What should you expect when you meditate? If you can't stop thinking when you try to sit quietly, remember that thoughts and distractions are normal. The goal is to observe your thoughts and simply let them pass quietly.

Think of your meditation session as if you are in a small boat, gently gliding down a river, a peaceful trip without much effort involved. There are many people, animals, and objects of interest along the shore. You make note of them, but you don't try to become involved with them; soon they move out of your range of vision and your consciousness.

Allow your thoughts a similar voyage. If you do get involved in an internal discussion, don't fight it. Acknowledge it, and then passively return to your mental focus and quiet breathing. Let your thoughts quietly float from your awareness.

As with learning any new skill, being able to meditate takes practice. Start with daily sessions of 5 to 10 minutes and slowly work up to 20-minute sessions. If you are afraid you'll fall asleep or lose track of time, set a quiet alarm so that you can fully relax, knowing that you can return to your usual routine when the time comes. But don't be too obsessed about the time. The idea is to encourage and train your body and mind to enter a state of relaxation when need be.

The Relaxation Response

Cardiologist Herbert Benson, M.D., first described the relaxation response in his 1975 book of the same name. While looking for a safe and effective treatment for patients with high blood pressure, Dr. Benson and his Harvard University team combined Western medical and scientific writings with Eastern spiritual traditions. The Boston medical group became convinced that lifestyle changes with an emphasis on relaxation could reverse the risk of heart attack, stroke, and stress-related symptoms such as insomnia.

The four basic elements necessary to elicit the positive physiological changes of the relaxation response are a quiet environment, a specific mental focus, such as repeating a word or gazing at a lighted candle, a passive and observing attitude, and a comfortable, relaxed position.

1. Sit in a chair or crosslegged on the floor.

2. Gently focus your attention on your breath. Breathe fully and deeply.

3. As you inhale, think "one," then exhale. Take another breath in, focus on the word "one," and exhale.

4. You can silently repeat other syllables or words, such as "peace," "relaxed," or "om" during meditation.

5. Continue meditating for 10 to 20 minutes.

This technique may feel awkward the first few times you try it. The challenge is to practice for 10 to 20 minutes, once or twice a day, for two weeks. Then evaluate your progress. Do you feel different after the two-week period? Are you more relaxed? If so, stick with it. The benefits of this stress management method can boost your sleep potential.

Revitalizing Yoga

Although historically rooted in Eastern religion, yoga has been popularized in North America as an exercise program that can both energize and relax. Yoga provides physical, psychological, and spiritual benefits. This versatile mind/body practice increases muscle flexibility, strength, and tone. It helps build physical immunity, corrects poor posture, and improves digestion and circulation. Practitioners also claim that yoga helps increase body awareness and relieves chronic stress patterns.

"There is a fullness of all things, even of sleep and of love."

HOMER

The University of Arizona's Integrative Medicine Clinic reports that yoga has been extremely useful in the treatment of stress-related disorders, including insomnia. The clinic also recommends yoga to help treat hypertension, arthritis, diabetes, chronic back pain, and digestive problems.

Guess who's going to yoga class? Recently, Susan, a married human-services professional with two children, started taking a class at the local wellness center. Rebecca, a college sophomore, signed up for Yoga 101 to fulfill her school's physical education requirement. And they are in fast-growing company. *Yoga Journal* estimates that approximately 12 million Americans now practice yoga regularly, a dramatic increase over the past six years.

If you would like to join this health-conscious crowd, choose a class offered by your local health club, community center, yoga studio, college, or HMO. The best way to learn yoga is to study with a qualified teacher. The feedback and hands-on instruction are keys to success.

In addition to beginner, intermediate, and advanced classes, many yoga teachers offer classes for people with special needs, such as seniors or women with breast cancer. Yoga centers may also advertise their style or school of yoga. Look for a beginner's-level hatha-style yoga class offered by the Kripalu or Integral schools. Power yoga, Ashtanga, and Iyengar classes are generally more strenuous. Consider attending a sample class or speak with the instructor to find a course suited for your skill level.

A typical beginner class starts with deep breathing and relaxation exercises. Next come the various body postures, called *asanas*, a series of basic to challenging stretches and positions done standing, sitting, or reclining. Gentle twists, back and side bends, and balancing postures may also be added. B. K. S. Iyengar, a yoga master, explained, "In each pose, there should be repose," so there needn't be any straining or competition. You hold each posture for as long as is comfortable within the limits of your body's flexibility. Class ends with a calming meditation.

Practicing yoga at any time of the day is calming. However, the American Yoga Association cautions that a full yoga workout in the evening may be too energizing and can interfere with sleep. But for those who are sleep deprived, a 15- to 30-minute session of gentle stretching and rhythmic breathing before bedtime can promote sleep.

Books and tapes with easy-to-follow instructions can help supplement your yoga practice at home. Some are specifically designed to help you sleep better. Before you purchase a tape, consider how much time you will be able to devote to yoga, as sessions generally range from 20 to 60 minutes.

Sleep-Inviting Music

The writer Diane Ackerman sensuously describes music as the perfume of hearing. In her book *A Natural History of the Senses*, she explains that "sounds thicken the sensory stew of our lives, and we depend on them to help us interpret, communicate with, and express the world around us." We may feel assaulted by the various noises we hear each day, but our moods can also be positively affected when we listen to uplifting or calming melodies.

Music therapy has been shown to benefit patients in hospitals and nursing homes. The healing power of music during diagnostic and surgical procedures, as well as in patients' rooms, helps alleviate pain, lessens depression and apprehension, calms the senses, and promotes sleep. It can actually reduce the amount of pain and of the sleep medication a patient needs.

"The rain plays a little sleep-song on our roof at night — And I love the rain."

LANGSTON HUGHES

Individuals with tension-related conditions benefit from musical stress reduction. In one study, 24 out of 25 people with insomnia dozed off more easily after listening to "new age" or classical music. Other studies show that listening to calm music can lessen anxiety and lower blood pressure and heart rate.

One important advantage of musical relaxation is that there is no training period and no technique to learn: The impact on

Harmonious Harp Music

Harpist Melissa Collins reports that according to Irish tradition, a master musician is one whose music can affect people in three important ways: make them laugh, make them cry, and put them to sleep. When Melissa plays music for hospice patients, they benefit from all of these effects. Listening to a tape of harp music before bed may also affect you emotionally and lull you to sleep.

the listener is immediate. Larry Dossey, M.D., a former director of a biofeedback clinic, notes that "music provide[s] the entry point for many people who otherwise [find] it impossible to enter relaxed states."

What type of music soothes and relaxes you? Easy listening, serene classics, light jazz? Don't know where to start? Don Campbell, author of *The Mozart Effect*, recommends specific passages of Mozart's music to "heal the body, strengthen the mind, and unlock the creative spirit." For inspired listening, order popular relaxation collections or recordings of nature sounds. Listen to soft, slow instrumental music as an accompaniment to soaking in the bath, practicing yoga, or simply getting ready to doze off. And remember: The transition to slumber will be facilitated by a sound system with a quiet, automatic shutoff.

Bodywork and Healing Hands

Bodywork comprises a number of techniques that involve touching or manipulating the body as a way to improve health and treat illness. These techniques can help alleviate stress-related conditions, including insomnia. Some methods work to subtly increase the energy flow in the body. Ancient Oriental traditions teach that many ailments are caused by a blockage in our bodies of the universal life energy, or *qi* (pronounced "chee"), which courses through all things. The objective is to unblock this energy to increase the body's natural healing capacities.

Massage

The most popular of the bodywork modalities, therapeutic massage promotes a sense of overall well-being and relaxation. Massage loosens tight muscles while lowering heart rate and blood pressure. It strengthens the immune system and helps the body release toxins. A massage also decreases the level of stress hormones in the body and increases the production of endorphins, the body's natural painkillers. It is especially good for sleeping problems due to stress, migraine headaches, and muscle and joint stiffness and pain.

Reflexology

Reflexology is based on the idea that the feet are minimaps of the body and internal organs. Reflexologists treat a wide variety of stress-related problems by pressing on various "reflex" or pressure points along the foot, which relieves symptoms elsewhere in the body. This healing technique can soothe the tension that causes sleeping problems.

Reiki

An ancient Japanese practice, *Reiki* is being used as an adjunct to conventional medicine in hospitals and hospices, as well as a treatment for the general public. Reiki practitioners gently place their hands in positions on a person's body, primarily near the seven energy centers known as *chakras,* to release energy blockages. Practitioners claim that *Reiki* speeds wound healing and postoperative recovery, and relieves pain, stress, anxiety, headaches, and insomnia.

"Night with her train of stars And her great gift of sleep."

WILLIAM ERNEST HENLEY

Acupuncture

Acupuncture is a branch of traditional Chinese medicine. This healing practice is also based on the belief that disease is caused by an energy imbalance in the body. An acupuncturist inserts extremely thin needles into a patient's body along the *meridians,* or energy pathways, stimulating energy flow. Although some pressure may be felt at the needle sites, patients generally report little or no discomfort.

Acupressure and Shiatsu

Acupressure, another ancient Chinese technique, and *Shiatsu,* a Japanese method, use finger pressure instead of needles to stimulate the body's natural healing abilities. This physical manipulation of the energy points clears the energy channels, releases tension, and treats disease.

You can also try stimulating acupressure points yourself. Gently press the specified point (see right), using your fingertips, steadily or with a small circular massage motion, for approximately one minute. After a break, you can repeat alternating pressure and breaks until you feel a sort of release. Beginners should not exceed 5 minutes on any one point.

How do you know whether you have the right spot? The pressure points "announce themselves with a feeling of tenderness, tingling, soreness, or minor discomfort," explains Michael Castleman in *Nature's Cures*.

Acupressure Points for Insomnia

1. **The hand.** With your palm facing up, find the juncture where the wrist meets the hand with the thumb of your other hand; rub just below the first crease of your wrist.

2. **The face.** Using the tips of your index and third fingers, apply pressure to the spot between your eyebrows, at the juncture of the bridge of your nose and your forehead.

3. **The back of the head.** Gently massage the pressure points at the indentation at the base of the skull on the back of the head; move outward an inch on both sides of the skull at the hairline.

8

Natural Remedies

There is a wide variety of natural remedies to aid the sleepless. For external use, herbal baths, compresses, and sleep pillows can gently lull you to sleep. Herbal teas, capsules, tinctures, and liquid extracts are stronger alternatives and are taken internally. Gentle homeopathic products and supplements are also available to treat insomnia. Health food stores and natural pharmacies stock many of these products.

Why herbs? Many people are turning away from chemical sedatives and tranquilizers because of their side effects. Within the past few years, an herbal renaissance has created an enormous increase in the use of alternative natural remedies.

Calming Chamomile

Chamomile (*Chamaemelum nobile* or *Matricaria recutita*) is the perfect choice to create a calm evening. Alexandra Stoddard, an interior decorator and prolific author of lifestyle books, was once filmed for an episode of the *Oprah* television show sitting on her bed sipping a cup of chamomile tea. Chamomile's pretty white flowers with yellow centers make a mild, relaxing beverage and are good in baths for sleepless adults and fussy babies.

The scent of chamomile tea is reminiscent of apple orchards. The herb has a relaxing effect on the nervous system, as it contains a compound that affects the same brain receptors as antianxiety drugs.

In addition to being a sleep aid, this wonderful herb relaxes the digestive system and

has traditionally been used to treat stomach-
aches, ulcers, and cramps. A cup of
chamomile tea may soothe evening heartburn
and indigestion. Remember Peter Rabbit? In
the children's book, Peter's mother served
him a cup of chamomile tea after his escape
from Mr. McGregor's garden. Many herbalists also recommend this herb as a colic
remedy for children.

Brewing Chamomile Tea

For a pleasant-tasting tea, steep chamomile
for no longer than five minutes, since it
becomes bitter if it's steeped too long.

In her delightful bath book *Water Magic*,
Mary Muryn describes how sharing an
evening with chamomile just may call you to
sleep. Following a chamomile steam facial,
put wet chamomile tea bags over your closed
eyes while you lie in a tub of chamomile-
infused water and sip a steaming cup of this
twilight tea. When this is accompanied by a

scented candle, soothing music, and an aromatic sleep pillow lightly scented with chamomile, almost anyone can be relaxed enough to fall asleep. (Wait until you are out of the bath and comfortably in bed, though!)

Chamomile Caution

As with all herb use, individual reactions may differ. Although the *PDR for Herbal Medicines* reports that chamomile has "a very weak potential for sensitization," some people, especially those with hay fever or other ragweed allergies, may experience an allergic reaction to the plant. The U.S. Federal Food and Drug Administration (FDA) lists chamomile as "generally regarded as safe."

Lavender Lullaby

Many of us long for luscious fields of fragrant French flowers. In lieu of a European vacation, we can be lulled to sleep by lounging in lavender (*Lavandula* spp.) for an evening. Among the attributes of this versatile herb is its ability to combat insomnia, nervousness, and headaches — and in such an aesthetic manner! The beauty of its deep purple-blue color, as well as its highly evocative scent, has made lavender a favorite for many centuries.

For the true lavender lover, there are never too many ways to use this fragrant and sedative plant. You can take a warm bath scented with lavender bath salts and wash with lavender soap. If you have a headache, add a lavender compress (a washcloth soaked in either the lavender bathwater or in strong lavender tea, wrung out, and then gently placed on your forehead). Keep the bathroom lights low and gently illuminate the space with some lavender-scented pillar candles.

A cup of sedative herbal tea flavored with organic dried lavender leaves is also delightful. To carry the scent into the bedroom, use a dryer sheet lightly sprinkled with lavender water after laundering your sheets. Or mist the bedroom with a lavender aromatherapy

"And still she slept an azure-lidded sleep, In blanched linen, smooth, and lavender'd"

JOHN KEATS

spray. Have your partner rub your back with a massage oil blended with lavender and sandalwood essential oils. And to ensure a tranquil night, the final touch is to rest your head on a sleep pillow laced with lavender.

Sleep Soundly Bath Salts

This recipe makes a wonderfully relaxing addition to your bath. Sedating bath salts packaged in pretty bottles also make lovely gifts.

⅔ cup baking soda
⅔ cup Epsom salts
⅔ cup sea salt
25–30 drops lavender essential oil

1. Thoroughly mix the baking soda, Epsom salts, sea salt, and lavender essential oil in a medium-sized nonporous bowl.
2. Cover the bowl with a cotton cloth and leave it to dry overnight.
3. Stir the mixture, breaking up any small chunks.

To use: Pour ½ cup of the bath salts into the tub as it is filling.

Other Herbs to Foster 40 Winks

There are many herbs renowned for their sleep-inducing and relaxing qualities. Although single herbs are available, many companies have created effective combination formulas. You can also try herbal teas, medicinal-strength tinctures (liquid extracts that preserve the herb's medicinal qualities in either an alcohol or a glycerin base), or capsules 30 to 45 minutes before bed.

California Poppy

California poppy *(Eschscholzia californica)* contains alkaloids with a sedative effect similar to that of the opiates codeine and morphine, but milder (and legal!). This herbal remedy helps reduce anxiety and promotes sleep. California poppy is often found in combination herbal sedative formulas.

Catnip

While it may stimulate your feline, catnip *(Nepeta cataria)* has the opposite effect on humans. This tasty and easy-to-grow cousin of mint makes a mild sedative tea as well as a nice addition to bath and sleep pillow formulas.

Hops

Hops *(Humulus lupulus)* were used by Native Americans for their sedative and digestive properties prior to their popular use as a beer-brewing ingredient. The cone-like flowers of the hop plant are strongly scented and somewhat bitter tasting. Hops should be used in a dried form, but the plant loses its effectiveness rapidly when stored, so buy small amounts. The FDA includes hops on its list of herbs that are "generally regarded as safe."

The herb has estrogenic properties that have effects on the body similar to those of female hormones. Because of this, hops should not be used by breast cancer patients. The hormonal effects seem to have advantages for menopausal women, however. Women's health educator and herbalist Susun Weed recommends hops tea as a powerful sleep enhancer and hormonal ally to women frequently awakened by night sweats. The sedative qualities of hops are best experienced when the dried flowers are used in an herbal tea or tincture mix, or to enhance herbal baths and sleep pillows.

Kava-Kava

A wonderful herbal remedy for mild to moderate anxiety, kava-kava *(Piper methysticum)* may also be an effective treatment for insomnia, studies show. Kava-kava helps produce a pleasant sense of relaxation and a sharpening of the senses while maintaining mental alertness. Pharmaceutical antianxiety medications are more sedating, and they slow down many mental and physical functions.

This ancient ceremonial and medicinal herb from the South Pacific islands has recently gained popularity in North America and is available in teas, capsules, extracts, and powdered form. Anecdotal accounts of kava-kava's worth as a sleep aid vary. Some people report that since the herb increases alertness, it can interfere with the ability to fall asleep.

It seems that the size and timing of the dose may affect its sleep-enhancing properties. After the initial alertness wears off, subsequent sleep can be deep and refreshing, so a small dose taken earlier in the day may produce alertness, then relaxation, and later sleep.

Lemon Balm

This herb is a delicious alternative to the bitter-tasting herbal sedatives. Lemon balm *(Melissa officinalis),* with a luscious citrus taste and aroma, helps relieve anxiety, insomnia, menstrual cramps, and mild digestive problems. In studies that used a combination of valerian extract and lemon balm, the effects were shown to be as powerful as those of pharmaceutical sleep medications. You can use lemon balm in teas, tinctures, baths, and sleep pillows.

Oatstraw

A cup of oatstraw tea? More familiar, of course, is the traditional nourishing breakfast grain. But herbalists Susun Weed and Deb Soule recommend oatstraw *(Avena sativa)* as a gentle, soothing relaxant. Oatstraw is thought to strengthen the nervous system and relieve pain. In the bath, oats soothe irritated skin.

Although it may not be strong enough for people with persistent sleep problems, a warm cup of oatstraw tea may relieve the occasional sleepless night caused by nervous tension, anxiety, or menopausal symptoms.

Passionflower

Passionflower *(Passiflora incarnata)* has been a favored sleep remedy since the days of the Aztecs and Incas. Currently, passionflower is a very popular insomnia remedy in Europe. Herbalist Kathi Keville recommends it for sleeplessness due to tight muscles or an overactive mind. On its own, passionflower is a mild sedative, but it combines well with valerian and is often used in combination tea, capsule, and tincture formulas.

Skullcap

Herbalists have much anecdotal evidence as to the merits of skullcap *(Scutellaria lateriflora)* as a relaxant and sedative. It has been used to treat insomnia and nervous disorders and as an antispasmodic for muscle cramps. Susun Weed claims, "Delicious, aromatic skullcap is my favorite painkiller and sleep inducer." Skullcap is often included in commercial combination sleep formulas.

St.-John's-Wort

Nicknamed the Prozac of Plants, St.-John's-wort *(Hypericum perforatum)* is an effective treatment for mild to moderate depression. Studies show that St.-John's-wort is as effective as many prescription antidepressants, with a much lower rate of side effects. This herbal remedy has been used extensively in Europe and its popularity has soared in the United States since the late 1990s.

If insomnia is associated with depression, St.-John's-wort may help. Since depression is a medical condition with possible serious consequences, consult a professional for correct diagnosis and treatment. Unlike many of the other herbal insomnia remedies, which can be taken on an as-needed basis, St.-John's-wort must be taken daily.

Initially, it can take four to six weeks before its benefits take effect.

St.-John's-wort may reduce the effectiveness of other medicines. The FDA has issued an advisory concerning the use of St.-John's-wort in combination with prescription medications, including anticancer drugs, heart medications, AIDS medicines, transplant rejection drugs, and some types of oral contraceptives. It may also magnify the effects of some anesthetic drugs. Consult a physician regarding the use of St.-John's-wort while taking any prescription medication, as well as prior to surgery.

Valerian

Valerian *(Valeriana officinalis)* is the premier herb to treat insomnia and stress. German studies have proved its benefits as a relaxant without sedative side effects. Included on the FDA's list of herbs "generally regarded as safe," valerian has also been used to treat menstrual cramps, backaches, headaches associated with the menstrual cycle, and intestinal upsets.

When valerian is paired with the more pleasant-tasting lemon balm, its strong odor is masked while its relaxing qualities are enhanced. Try the combination in liquid extracts or capsules. (*Note:* In a small percentage of users, valerian is stimulating rather than relaxing; discontinue its use if this is the case.) Dr. Andrew Weil cautions that people with impaired kidney or liver function not take valerian except under a physician's supervision.

Nonwestern Herbs

Practitioners of Chinese medicine recommend jujube seeds *(Ziziphus jujuba)* as a treatment for insomnia. Since most of the research concerning the safety and efficacy of jujube has been done in China and is not yet translated, this remedy should be used only after consulting a specialist in traditional Chinese medicine. Jujube is available in pill form in combination with other Chinese herbs.

Some practitioners of Ayurvedic medicine, a branch of traditional Indian medicine, recommend ashwagandha *(Withania somnifera)*, an ancient herbal remedy, to treat insomnia. Also known as "Indian ginseng," ashwagandha provides complementary energizing and calming benefits. The standardized extract can be mixed with warm milk for a soothing bedtime tisane.

Other Ayurvedic practitioners recommend the topical use of herbal oils to encourage sleep while nourishing the hair. Hair brushing or scalp massage with oils infused with bhringaraj *(Eclipta alba)* and gotu kola *(Centella asiatica)* is said to calm the mind and promote sound sleep.

Herbal Teas

Mark Blumenthal, executive director of the American Botanical Council, eloquently described teatime's appeal when he said, "Drinking tea can take you into another dimension, another time and place, a time when things were slower, gentler, warmer, cozier. It can be a gastronomic form of meditation."

To ease into sleep, add some soothing and sedating herbal tea to your evening ritual. It provides a perfect antidote to a rushed and overly full day. Put your feet up, sip your tea, and listen to soft music. If you can't find seclusion in the more public areas of your busy household, take a cup of tea into your bedroom. Close the door and drink the tea slowly during a quiet 20-minute period.

On busy days, you can just drop a tea bag into any old mug, fill it with hot water, wait three minutes, wring out the tea bag with a spoon, and drink a quick "cuppa." But good equipment and know-how will make the tea-making experience more pleasurable. Here's how to do it right:

1. Fill your teapot with hot tap water. Let it warm up the pot while you bring cold water to a boil for your tea.

2. Empty the teapot and measure in the loose tea. Use a teaspoon of dried herb or a tablespoon of fresh herb for each cup of boiling water.

3. Pour the boiling water over the herbs. Cover the teapot and steep the herbs

for 5 to 10 minutes, or longer for medicinal strength.

4. Strain out the herbs and serve the tea hot. Add milk if desired. If you are drinking the tea before bedtime, use a light hand with the sweetener, as it can be stimulating.

Sleep Soundly Herbal Tea

This sedative beverage has a mild citrus flavor.

> 1 cup dried chamomile flowers
> 1 cup dried lemon balm
> ½ cup dried catnip
> ½ cup dried oatstraw
> ¼ cup dried valerian or hops (optional)

1. Mix the herbs well and store the blend in an airtight jar.
2. Use 1 teaspoon of the blend for each cup of tea.

Herbal Baths

Add herbs to your bath to enhance its natural stress-reducing and sleep-inducing qualities. You can use sedating scents in the form of essential oils, bath salts, or herbal bath bags.

Sleep Soundly Bath Bags

This recipe includes a beautiful bouquet of pleasantly scented, sleep-promoting herbs. Oatmeal is a great skin-softening addition, especially during the dry winter months.

1 cup dried chamomile flowers
1 cup dried lavender flowers
1 cup oatmeal (optional)
½ cup dried hops
½ cup dried rose petals

1. Combine all of the ingredients.
2. Place ½ cup of the mixture in the center of a piece of permeable fabric and tie it closed. (Small drawstring bags in cotton or muslin work well, as do thin washcloths.)
3. When running the bath, loop the tie over the faucet so the water runs through the bag as the tub fills.

Herbal Sleep Pillows

Herbal pillows, or "sleep bags," have a long history. Hildegard von Bingen, a 12th-century German abbess and herbalist, recommended using herb-filled sachets for better sleep. Sleep pillows were widely used during the Colonial period to induce sleep and promote healing for the sick.

At home or while traveling, sleep pillows make wonderful companions. Some bed-and-breakfast owners keep optional scented pillows around for their herbal-minded patrons. And many travelers stash a small herbal sleep sachet in their carry-on luggage to soothe their senses during plane trips and to sweeten nights spent in stuffy hotel rooms.

Sedating Scents

The most important consideration in making an herbal sleep pillow is choosing the right mix of sedating scents to help the recipient relax and sleep. Start with a combination of dried lavender, chamomile, lemon balm, hops, and rose petals. Author Jim Long provides a number of recipes for

"The night comes on, And sleep upon this little world of ours, Spreads out her sheltering, healing wings."

ELIZA LEE FOLLEN,
WRITER AND POET

fragrant dream and sleep pillows in his beautifully illustrated book *Making Herbal Dream Pillows*.

Keep in mind that not all relaxing herbs have pleasant aromas or associations for the sleeper. For example, many find hops, a wonderfully calming herb, too bitter smelling. But combined with sweeter scents, such as lavender and rose, it increases the sleep-inducing properties of the pillow while its smell is toned down.

Be aware that some companies sell "dream pillows" that are intended to induce more vivid dreams for the user. These are not good choices for the sleepless searching for a calm night.

Making Sleep Pillows

The other practical considerations when making herbal pillows are the size and shape of the pillow, the fabric with which it's covered, and its ability to be cleaned.

A small pillow that is flat and not plump is recommended. When it's placed between your usual pillow and the pillowcase, its sweet, calming aroma will be released each time you turn your head during the night. The sizes of sleep pillows usually range from a small 4-inch square to a larger 9- by 11-inch rectangle.

There are many great fabric textures, weights, and designs to choose from. For durability, you can make an inner muslin pillow filled with herbs and sheathed in a detachable, washable cover. Consider using a fanciful fabric with a celestial pattern or a calming shade of blue to match the evening dream theme.

You can fill your pillow with herbs alone or shape it first with cotton batting or a synthetic pillow stuffing. It is generally cheaper to make pillows with a type of filler. Sprinkle one to two tablespoons of herb mix between thin layers of the stuffing. This method also assures a softer pillow and lessens the chance of having leaves or twigs stick through the pillow cover.

Pillows recommended as sleep aids for children are often filled with one herb — usually dill, chamomile, or catnip. These three herbs are purported to gently lull a child to sleep and to deter nightmares.

Sleep Soundly Pillow Mix

This is a sweet but potent combination of sedative herbs. Adjust the proportions according to your personal preference and the availability of herbs.

4 parts dried lavender flowers
2 parts dried hops
2 parts dried rose petals
1 part dried chamomile
1 part dried lemon balm

Aromatherapy

Do you stop and smell the roses? Be aware of which aromas surround you. Does a coworker wear a signature cologne? Are you conscious of the fragrance of your soap and shampoo? Does your house smell of fresh flowers, cleansers, baby powder, or food?

Subconsciously, various aromas can please or annoy you. Scents affect your mood and your health; they can even affect your ability to sleep. The best way to enhance your sleep with scents is to use soothing essential oils.

Aromatherapy is the practice of using essential oils to comfort and heal, and there is a long history, particularly in Europe, of their medicinal use. The emotional and physiological effects of essential oils go beyond personal association. Each of the oils, extracted from a specific herb or flower, has its own unique healing qualities. These highly concentrated oils can be absorbed into the body through the skin or through the olfactory bulb in the nose.

Essential oils can provide a sensuous solution to your sleep problems. Scientific and anecdotal accounts feature lavender essential oil as the primary choice to treat insomnia. Purchase it, or any of the other

Calming Essential Oils

- ★ Bergamot
- ★ Chamomile
- ★ Clary sage
- ★ Lavender
- ★ Lemon balm
- ★ Orange
- ★ Rose
- ★ Sandalwood
- ★ Sweet marjoram
- ★ Ylang-ylang

calming and relaxing essential oils, singly or in combination.

To restore restful sleep, try using essential oils diluted in massage oils, bath products, facial steams, footbaths, and scented pillows. Mist your bedroom with a mellow mood-enhancing room spray. Commercial room diffusers provide a gentle continuous aromatic vapor. Compresses are

Be Careful

Do not confuse essential oils with their synthetic counterparts, which are often sold for hobby or craft purposes. The synthetic oils do not provide the healing qualities of the pure essences. Since essential oils are highly concentrated, do not use them at full strength.

There are rarely problems reported with essential oils, but those prone to migraines, asthma, and skin allergies shouldn't use them. Never ingest essential oils unless under the care of a certified aromatherapist.

also helpful for insomnia due to tension headaches.

For the traveler, aromatherapy can provide relief from stress and jet lag. You can carry homemade "smelling salts" to calm you during a long flight. Combine 5 to 10 drops of a relaxing essential oil with 2 tablespoons of salt and pour the mixture into a small bottle. Or put 1 to 3 drops of oil on a cotton ball and place it in a plastic bag.

Sleep Soundly Room Spray

Use this mild sedating mist to freshen your bedroom or spray it directly on your sheets and pillows and you'll learn to associate sleep with its calming scent.

1 cup distilled water
2 tablespoons vodka (optional, as a preservative)
9 drops lavender essential oil
6 drops bergamot essential oil
3 drops sandalwood essential oil

1. Combine all of the ingredients.
2. Shake the mixture well before each use and don't spray it on furniture.

Homeopathy

Billed as a safe and effective alternative to conventional medicine, homeopathy is a medical system developed more than 200 years ago that remains more popular in parts of Europe than it does in the United States.

In *Healing Homeopathic Remedies,* Nancy Bruning and Corey Weinstein, M.D., explain, "Homeopathy holds that symptoms represent the body's best efforts to heal itself, and therefore, they should not be suppressed. Unlike conventional drugs, homeopathic remedies stimulate our own innate powers to heal ourselves — without adding any harmful side effects." Several homeopathic remedies are effective for treating anxiety, overstimulation, and emotional upset that can lead to sleep problems.

Arsenicum

Arsenicum is used when the cause of insomnia is fear or anxiety. It helps people who are generally restless after midnight, and who feel chilly and want extra blankets.

Homeopathic Highlights

Below are the major principles that form the basis of the homeopathic medical system.

1. The Law of Similars states that "like cures like." Homeopathic remedies are made from extremely diluted substances. When given in large doses to healthy people, the substances cause a specific set of symptoms; the dilute homeopathic remedy relieves those same symptoms in people who are ill.

2. Practitioners treat the totality of symptoms. Remedies are selected based on an individual patient's symptoms and temperament, as well as the interaction between the two.

3. The minimum dose rule holds that remedies should be given in infinitesimal doses. Practitioners believe that the extreme dilution of homeopathic remedies makes them more potent.

Coffea

Coffea treats insomnia owing to overstimulation of the body or mind due to excitement or bad news. As its name suggests, it is good for those who stay awake because of coffee consumption.

Ignatia

Ignatia is for the person whose sleeplessness is caused by emotional upset or grief, who dreads not being able to sleep, and who may have nightmares.

Nux vomica

Nux vomica is recommended for sleep problems caused by excessive intake of coffee, alcohol, or other drugs; or food; or from mental overexertion. The remedy is especially suited for people who sleep fitfully and wake around 2 to 3 A.M.

Pulsatilla

Pulsatilla is for those who can't fall asleep until after midnight and wake up a few hours later, often with recurring thoughts that are like a "broken record."

Using Homeopathic Remedies

Homeopathic remedies are available in most health food stores and natural pharmacies. Place the small pellets under your tongue to dissolve; do not eat anything for 15 minutes before or after taking the remedy. Strong substances, such as coffee, chocolate, or peppermint, may negate the benefits of homeopathic treatments; this is especially true for homeopathic insomnia remedies. Follow the package insert for specific instructions. For long-term problems, consult a trained homeopath.

Soporific Supplements

There are a number of dietary supplements touted as sleep potions. Some of these, sold primarily in health food stores and natural pharmacies, are synthesized forms of naturally occurring body chemicals, such as hormones and amino acids.

A few have been the focus of late-breaking news and some are still in the center of controversy. Proponents maintain that these supplements are good alternatives for enhancing sleep. Critics point out that their long-term effects have not yet been adequately studied and some serious questions have been raised concerning their safety.

Melatonin

A naturally occurring hormone, melatonin is secreted by the pineal gland in the brain. Since its production rises at night and falls during the day, it has been dubbed "the hormone of darkness," affecting our internal body clock and sleep cycles.

Many health claims have been made concerning the use of synthetic melatonin as a dietary supplement. Experts concur that melatonin is okay for occasional use to treat insomnia, but that it is better used as a remedy to prevent or reduce the symptoms of jet lag.

Based on the premise that our natural melatonin levels decrease as we age, the supplement is also hyped as a potential

"Some say that gleams of a remoter world Visit the soul in sleep."

PERCY BYSSHE
SHELLEY

"fountain of youth." However, a recent Harvard University study has raised doubts about whether or not melatonin levels decline with age.

In addition, the results or a number of studies concerning the effectiveness of melatonin supplementation for insomnia differ, as does the anecdotal evidence. In a survey conducted by *Consumer Reports*, respondents judged melatonin to be a less effective treatment for insomnia than exercise, prescription drugs, and over-the-counter medications.

The University of California, Berkeley, Wellness Letter reports that melatonin helps people fall asleep faster, but it may not help them stay asleep and can produce a "hangover" and drowsiness the next day.

The long-term effects of melatonin are not known. Research continues to study its efficacy as a sleep aid. Due to melatonin's connection to our daily light cycles, encouraging studies are being conducted with shift workers and blind people with sleep problems. Scientists also say that melatonin is a powerful antioxidant that may protect us against chronic diseases. Ongoing research is needed to prove its benefits.

Tryptophan

Tryptophan, an amino acid, is a precursor to serotonin, a brain chemical involved in the regulation of sleep and mood, and to melatonin, an important sleep hormone. Up until the late 1980s, supplemental tryptophan was recommended as a potent insomnia remedy. Peter Hauri, M.D., and Shirley Linde, M.D., report in their book *No More Sleepless Nights* that there are at least 25 studies suggesting that taking tryptophan in the evening helps about half of insomniacs.

The FDA banned the sale of tryptophan supplements in 1990 after it was found that a contaminated batch caused an outbreak of eosinophilia-myalgia (EMS) syndrome. The disease affected more than 1500 people and was the cause of at least 38 deaths.

Tryptophan is available as a supplement in other countries. Since the EMS outbreak was a result of a faulty manufacturing process and not caused by a problem with the pure product, some people believe that tryptophan should again be made available to the public.

5-HTP

A naturally occurring compound, 5-HTP (5-hydroxytryptophan) is directly related to tryptophan and also boosts serotonin levels. Supplements are synthesized from the seeds of *Griffonia simplicifolia.* Dr. Andrew Weil reports that 5-HTP supplements have been used for decades in Europe as an approved treatment for depression and sleep problems.

In August 1998, the FDA confirmed the presence of impurities in some 5-HTP products marketed as dietary supplements. No toxicity or specific illnesses have been reported. As of this writing, 5-HTP supplements are available, though the FDA continues to monitor these products and remains "concerned."

Using Herbs Safely

Herbs can provide a wonderful, all-natural remedy for sleeplessness. However, like all substances used for medicinal purposes, herbs must be administered with caution to be both safe and effective. When you use herbal remedies, here are some ideas to keep in mind:

★ The goal is to achieve unmedicated, restful sleep. Herbal remedies, especially ones used internally, are for short-term or intermittent use only.

★ The fact that herbs are "natural" doesn't mean you don't have to follow precautions when taking them. Follow recommended doses; more is not better.

★ Do not take herbal sedatives while pregnant or nursing, except after consultation with your health-care provider.

★ Alternate herbal sleep remedies; there is a chance of building up a tolerance with continuous use of any one.

★ Start with the gentler herbs and remedies, such as a cup of chamomile tea and an herbal bath, before moving on to the stronger remedies.

★ Check with your health-care practitioner before combining any medicinal herb with prescription medications. Do not use calming herbs while taking tranquilizers, sedatives, antidepressants, alcohol, or other sleep medications.

★ Get advice from a naturopath, an herbalist, or a physician knowledgeable about complementary medicine.

★ Read about the remedies and lifestyle changes you are anticipating. Join or start an herbal study group.

★ Most herbal sedatives should be taken 30 to 45 minutes before bedtime. Follow the label's instructions.

9

When Self-Help Doesn't Help

Has your sleep problem gone on for far too long? Chronic sleeplessness causes emotional drain and physical ailments. Fatigue and irritability can cloud your judgment, making it difficult to assess your options and make an informed decision.

The short-term use of sleep medications can help. You may want to consult a health-care provider, who can assist you in finding the best path to sound sleep.

When to Seek Professional Help

Chronic medical problems often don't respond to self-help remedies. If your sleep problem is persistent or periodically recurs, seek conventional medical assessment and treatment. A family physician or general practitioner can prescribe sleeping pills or refer you to a sleep clinic for further evaluation. The sleep associations listed in the resource section (see page 181) can provide you with valuable information and referrals.

Prescription Medications

The issue of prescription sleep medications is complex and controversial. More than five billion doses of tranquilizers and sleeping pills are dispensed yearly in the United States. The medicines vary in strength, duration, and potential side effects.

Over-the-Counter Remedies

Some people find relief from over-the-counter (OTC) sleep remedies. When using OTCs to treat transient insomnia, be sure to check product labels for their ingredients and cautions. Acetaminophen is an ingredient in some OTC sleep remedies; continual use of acetaminophen is associated with anemia, kidney damage, and ulcers.

Many OTC sleep remedies also contain antihistamines, which can cause drowsiness, dry mouth, impotence, dizziness, blurred vision, and sometimes insomnia. Studies show that older adults are more likely to experience confusion, irritability, nervousness, and nightmares while taking these medications. They may also interfere with a brain chemical crucial for memory. Christiane Northrup, M.D., emphasizes, "Repeatedly taking OTC sleep remedies or cold remedies that contain antihistamines can result in memory problems and confusion over time."

Sleeping pills can increase your level of tolerance, necessitating higher doses to achieve the same effect. Some sleep medications may also cause a rebound effect, worsening the insomnia when the medication is discontinued. Sleeping pills can cause dangerous interactions with other medications and should never be taken with alcohol, sedatives, or tranquilizers.

Sleep educators recommend the judicious use of sleeping pills for the symptomatic relief of temporary insomnia. For many patients, sleep medications provide the only way to break the frustrating cycle of sleeplessness and fatigue. One troubled sleeper, who agrees, describes her situation: "After having trouble sleeping for many weeks, it felt like I had stepped over a line. Nothing worked. I needed medical help to stop my exhaustion and my fear of not sleeping! Only after a week or so of medicated sleep did sedative baths, herbal teas, and meditation help at all. First, I just had to sleep, and then I needed to relearn how to sleep better without any drugs."

Ask your physician about the shorter-acting sleeping pills that have recently come onto the market. These drugs travel through the body faster and are less apt to cause daytime grogginess. The shorter-acting drugs seem most useful for those who have difficulty falling asleep, but, since their effects last for approximately four hours, they can also be taken if the problem is waking up in the middle of the night unable to fall back to sleep. After a few nights of refreshing sleep, you may then choose to complement your treatment with natural methods.

Use sleep medications only on a short-term basis and at the lowest effective dose and wean yourself from the drug gradually. Talk with your pharmacist or a health-care professional before starting any new medication.

> "Sleep that knits up the ravell'd sleave [sic] of care, The death of each day's life, sore labor's bath, Balm of hurt minds, great nature's second course, Chief nourisher in life's feast."
>
> WILLIAM SHAKESPEARE

Conclusion: It's Time to Say Good Night

> "Blessings on him that first invented sleep! It covers a man, thoughts and all, like a cloak; it is meat for the hungry, drink for the thirsty, heat for the cold, and cold for the hot."
>
> MIGUEL DE CERVANTES SAAVEDRA

While in line at a bookstore café during a recent afternoon, I overheard an interesting conversation between two women. One woman, who ordered a glass of juice, asked her friend, "Aren't you having problems sleeping at night? Why don't you skip that espresso?"

The java lover responded, "Well, since I'm probably not going to sleep tonight anyway, why deprive myself of one of my little pleasures?" Why, indeed?

Sometimes sleep challenges are symptomatic of underlying issues; other times a few small changes will help restore sound sleep. For example, when a colleague was experiencing insomnia following a recent job change, he was concerned that his sleep problem might indicate that the career switch had been a mistake.

Discussion revealed that he really did like his new position but that some important circumstances had changed. Not only did he now begin work earlier each day, but the new job also moved him from a previously well-lighted office to a dim basement one. A combination of herbal sedatives and early morning light helped him return to a satisfying sleep pattern.

For some people, a lack of sleep clouds judgment, magnifying their problems. This became evident during my work with a psychotherapy client who was experiencing anxiety and insomnia. Initially, the woman was intent on making a major life change to alleviate her nervousness.

However, after learning relaxation techniques and following sleep hygiene guidelines, including allowing herself ample sleep time, she experienced relief and appreciation of her current situation. Although the client wanted to make some changes in her life, when adequately rested she no longer believed that drastic measures were necessary.

By itself, extra sleep won't solve your problems, but it can provide you with the energy and fresh perspective for finding solutions. Sound sleep creates a foundation for a healthy physical, psychological, and spiritual life. The choices and changes we make can have a tremendous effect on our ability to sleep. We may need to make some sacrifices, but I believe that the trade-offs are well worth the rest and renewal that they will provide.

What do you need to do to experience more of this sweet pleasure? How would your life improve if you got more and better sleep? Think about it. Better yet, using the suggestions you've read here, sleep on it.

"To all, to each, a fair goodnight, And pleasing dreams, and slumbers light!"

Sir Walter Scott

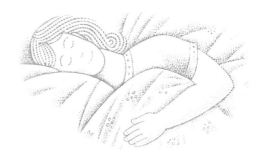

Resources

Author Contact

BHpurple@aol.com

Organizations

**American Sleep Apnea
Association**
1424 K Street NW, Suite 302
Washington, DC 20005
(202) 293-3650
www.sleepapnea.org

**National Center on Sleep
Disorders Research**
NIH Information Center
P.O. Box 30105
Bethesda, Maryland 20892
(301) 592-8573
www.nhlbisupport.com/sleep

National Sleep Foundation
1522 K Street NW, Suite 500
Washington, DC 20005
(202) 347-3471
www.sleepfoundation.org

Herbal Suppliers

Frontier Co-op Herbs
3021 78th Street
P.O. Box 299
Norway, IA 52318
(800) 717-4372
www.frontierherb.com

Jean's Greens
119 Sulfur Spring Road
Norway, NY 13416
(888) 845-TEAS
www.jeansgreens.com

Mountain Rose Herbs
20818 High Street
North San Juan, CA 95960
(800) 879-3337
www.botanical.com/mt.rose

Audiotapes and Videotapes

Living Arts
2434 Main Street
Santa Monica, CA 90405
(800) 2-LIVING
www.gaiam.com

Sounds True
P.O. Box 8010
Boulder, Colorado 80306
(800) 333-9185
www.soundstrue.com

Yoga Enterprises Inc.
30 Lincoln Plaza, Suite 27
New York, NY 10023
(888) YES-YOGA
www.stretch.com

Index

Other Storey Titles You Will Enjoy

7 Simple Steps to Unclutter Your Life, by Donna Smallin. For readers who yearn for more balance in their lives, this book offers hundreds of tips and ideas for enhancing physical, emotional, and spiritual well-being while creating a simpler, less stressful lifestyle. 176 pages. Paperback. ISBN 1-58017-237-7.

365 Ways to Relax Mind, Body & Soul, by Barbara L. Heller. From simple, uplifting thoughts to soothing exercises to relaxing foods and diet advice, this book offers effective ways to beat stress and promote relaxation in a fun, gift-book format. 384 pages. Paperback. ISBN 1-58017-332-2.

Feeling Fabulous Every Day: 250 Simple and Natural Ways to Achieve Spiritual, Emotional, and Physical Well-Being, by Stephanie Tourles. This guide to feeling and looking great includes hundreds of tips for eating well, living a balanced life, and taking care of yourself. 192 pages. Paperback. ISBN 1-58017-313-6.

The Healing Aromatherapy Bath, by Margó Valentine Lazzara. Combining aromatherapy with hypnotherapy, this hands-on approach to mind/body healing offers essential-oil formulas to use in the bath along with guided imagery and meditation exercises. 160 pages. Paperback. ISBN 1-58017-197-4.

Herbs for Reducing Stress and Anxiety, by Rosemary Gladstar. One of America's foremost herbalists provides concise, simple, and practical information for using herbs to relieve stress and anxiety. 96 pages. Paperback. ISBN 1-58017-155-9.

These books and other Storey books are available
at your bookstore, farm store, garden center,
or directly from Storey Books, Schoolhouse Road,
Pownal, Vermont 05261, or by calling 1-800-441-5700.
Or visit our Web site at www.storeybooks.com